MASTERING THE ART OF LETTING GO

OF EMOTIONAL PAIN & TOXIC RELATIONSHIPS

Self-Love, Self-Acceptance
& Finding Your Inner Peace
for Teens & Young Adults

 JEROME PURYEAR MD

Legal Notice
The information contained within this book is provided for educational and informational purposes only, and no reliance is to be placed on its contents. Effort has been made to present accurate, reliable, and current information; however, no warranties of any kind, expressed or implied, are made regarding its completeness, accuracy, or suitability for any particular purpose.

The author and publisher are not rendering medical, legal, financial, psychological, or other professional advice or services. Readers should consult a licensed professional before applying any strategies, techniques, or recommendations described herein.

By reading this book, you agree that under no circumstances shall the author or publisher be liable for any direct or indirect loss, injury, or damages arising from the use or misuse of the material contained within, including but not limited to errors, omissions, or inaccuracies.

All trademarks, product names, and company names mentioned are the property of their respective owners and are used for identification purposes only.

Eternaverse Publishing books may be purchased in bulk for business, educational, or promotional use.
For information, please contact your local bookseller or
Eternaverse Publishing at SpecialMarkets@eternaversepublishing.com.

Eternaverse Publishing authors are available for speaking engagements.
To find out more, email SpeakerBureau@eternaversepublishing.com.

*For every young person who has ever felt
the weight of the world on their shoulders,
who has carried pain that wasn't theirs to keep,
and who is ready to choose their own peace.*

*This book is a love letter to your resilience
and a guide back to your authentic self.*

HELP SPREAD THE WORD!

If this book has helped you **release an old hurt**,
set a healthy boundary, or simply **find
a little more hope on a hard day**,
I'd be so grateful if you'd leave a review on Amazon.

Scan the QR code below
to share your reflection.

Your words matter—your story can help someone else
begin their healing journey.

Each review helps others discover this work,
and reminds other teens and young adults
that they're not alone on the path to peace.

**Your light inspires healing.
Your voice builds hope.**
Keep honoring your journey—
I'm rooting for you every step of the way.

CONTENTS

Letter to the Reader

To the brave souls embarking on this journey,

Thank you. Thank you for choosing this book and, most importantly, for choosing yourself.

For over two decades, I've worked as a diagnostic and interventional radiologist. My days are spent looking at images of the human body—seeing the intricate details of bones, organs, and tissues. I've learned to spot anomalies, identify problems, and guide interventions to fix them. I see pain in its physical form every single day.

But I've come to realize that some of the most profound pain isn't visible on an X-ray or an MRI. It's the silent, emotional ache that so many of us carry—especially during our teenage and young adult years. It's the weight of a toxic relationship, the sting of a thoughtless word, the burden of expectations, and the lingering pain that holds us back.

I wrote this book because I believe the skills I've honed in my professional life—identifying the problem, understanding its source, and taking action to heal—are just as critical for our emotional well-being. This book is my way of translating those years of experience into a practical guide for you.

This isn't just a book of theory; it's a toolkit. It's a collection of practical exercises, reflections, and even meditations to help you develop the skills you need to navigate this part of your life. My hope is that you'll see it as a safe space where you can learn to:

- Understand and manage your emotions instead of being overwhelmed by them
- Build unbreakable boundaries that protect your peace
- Identify and navigate relationships with clarity and confidence
- Discover the power of self-love and self-care as foundational tools for a happy life
- Cultivate a growth mindset so that pain becomes a teacher, not a prison

This journey won't always be easy, but it will be worth it. The goal isn't to erase your past or pretend the pain never happened. It's about learning from it, letting go of what no longer serves you, and making space for a future filled with joy, purpose, and healthy relationships.

You have the power to heal and thrive. This book is just a starting point. I'm honored to be a part of your journey toward a life of emotional freedom.

I know how brave you are for seeking a path to lighter days. This isn't just a book; it's a companion for your journey toward emotional freedom. Every exercise, strategy, and word inside was written with compassion for what you're going through and designed to be a practical toolkit for untangling the heavy feelings and relationships that hold you back.

Your peace is the priority. Let's begin.

With gratitude,

Jerome Puryear, MD

Introduction

I remember the day I finally let go of my fear of failure. It felt as though I had been carrying a heavy backpack filled with years of self-doubt and unrealistic expectations, and I was finally able to set it down. Standing in front of the mirror, I took a deep breath and said, "You are enough, just as you are." That moment wasn't just an affirmation; it marked the beginning of a change—a catalyst that initiated a journey of personal development, emotional strength, and self-acceptance. This book is the result of that process, and I am excited to share it with you.

The world we live in is brimming with expectations. Pressures from family, friends, colleagues, and society often create an overwhelming sense of who we should be and how we should measure success. On top of that, the expectations we impose on ourselves frequently magnify this weight, making it difficult to feel at peace. Have you ever tried to meet these demands only to feel drained, frustrated, or lost? Many of us experience this struggle, yet there is another path forward. It involves learning to navigate these pressures and finding the strength to define your life on your own terms.

Consider a moment we've all faced: scrolling through social media and coming across an image of someone living a life that seems perfect. Perhaps it's a friend on an incredible vacation, celebrating a promotion, or achieving a milestone you haven't yet reached. That familiar pang of doubt surfaces, whispering, *Why not me? What am I doing wrong?* This book offers tools to help shift your mindset in moments like these. Instead of letting those emotions take hold, you will learn to pause, reflect, and release the comparisons that weigh you down.

Practical strategies are at the heart of this book. These tools will help you understand and manage your emotions, freeing you from the grip of doubt and fear. You'll discover techniques to build self-awareness and uncover the deeper roots of your feelings and behaviors. This understanding is the foundation for meaningful change.

This journey is open to all. Whether you are a teenager learning to manage the challenges of growing up, a young adult stepping into new phases of independence, a parent supporting your children, or an educator searching for ways to uplift others, the insights here can make a difference. The challenges of self-doubt and comparison touch every stage of life, but so do the opportunities for growth and self-compassion.

Emotional challenges are often seen as deeply personal, but they are also universal. Experiences of fear, loneliness, or inadequacy are not unique to one person; they are part of the human condition. These feelings don't define our value but instead offer opportunities to learn and grow. This book offers practical strategies, engaging examples, and insightful exercises to help you turn emotional barriers into pathways leading to a richer, more rewarding life.

Emotional intelligence is important for personal development. By understanding and regulating your emotions, you can face life's challenges with purpose rather than defaulting to impulsive reactions. Heightened emotional awareness enhances your relationships, sharpens decision-making, and enriches your sense of purpose. Rather than shunning emotions, you will learn to welcome them, recognizing their role in driving both personal and relational development.

Growth rarely follows a straight path. The process involves moments of discovery, setbacks, and progress. Sometimes, it requires bold actions, such as making significant life changes. Other times, breakthroughs come in quieter moments, such as choosing to pause during a stressful situation or practicing kindness toward yourself after making a mistake. These moments, big and small, shape the journey.

Throughout this book, you'll encounter stories and examples from others who have faced similar struggles. Each journey highlights a unique path to healing and self-discovery. There is no single way to reach emotional freedom, and that is the beauty of this process. Individual experiences and perspectives enrich the understanding of what it means to grow emotionally and embrace authenticity.

The strategies in this book are not abstract ideas but practical tools you can apply to your everyday life. With mindfulness exercises and techniques for managing stress, these tools are designed to meet you at your level and help you move forward. Each chapter builds on the last, providing actionable steps to help you lift emotional burdens, strengthen your resilience, and nurture a deeper sense of self-worth.

Reaching out for help is an essential part of the journey. Turning to trusted friends, family, or professionals shows both courage and a genuine desire to grow. In a world that often glorifies independence, we sometimes forget how much strength lies in connection. Sharing your challenges and victories with others deepens relationships and adds richness to life. Community support provides a safe space where healing and transformation can genuinely occur.

This book isn't about promising a life without challenges—it's an invitation to see those challenges in a new light. Difficult moments can become opportunities to discover more about yourself and tap into your inner strength. As you explore the tools and stories in these pages, you'll start to uncover your unique path to emotional resilience and fulfillment.

Each chapter of this book is crafted to offer insights and exercises that help you move forward with confidence, release self-doubt, embrace vulnerability, and align with your true self. The aim isn't perfection but progress—building a life that reflects your values, strengths, and aspirations.

Beginning this journey requires courage, as it involves looking inward, facing fears, and cultivating self-compassion. Yet, the rewards are impactful: a sense of freedom, deeper connections, and a renewed sense of self-worth. With each lesson and exercise, you'll uncover your strength and potential, growing into someone who faces challenges with courage, celebrates their unique gifts, and lives with purpose and joy. This journey is about self-discovery, growth, and finding emotional freedom, providing you with the tools to create a life full of purpose and genuine connection.

CHAPTER 1

Understanding Emotional Burdens

Acknowledging our emotional scars is the first step toward healing the invisible wounds that hold us back.

We all carry emotional burdens, even if we can't always see them. These invisible weights—guilt, anxiety, unresolved conflicts, and the expectations placed on us—can quietly shape our lives in powerful ways. They can hold us back, keeping us from reaching our potential or finding true peace. Whether it's self-doubt stopping us from taking a chance or the pressure to meet others' standards dictating our choices, these burdens influence how we see ourselves and interact with the world. Recognizing what we're carrying is the first step toward letting go and moving forward.

In this chapter, we will take a closer look at our emotional burdens and explore practical ways to start lightening this load that impacts our lives. Some burdens arise from within, such as harsh self-criticism, while others stem from external sources like family expectations and societal pressures. Both can weigh us down in ways we may not recognize, but understanding them can reveal how they shape our thoughts, actions, and relationships. Through reflection, mindfulness, and honest conversations with ourselves, we can uncover what's holding us back and begin to address it. This journey isn't just about identifying our struggles—it's about turning them into opportunities for growth, resilience, and strength. Together, we'll find ways to overcome these challenges and move closer to the peace and empowerment we all deserve.

IDENTIFYING EMOTIONAL BURDENS

Emotional burdens often operate in silence, yet their impact is significant, holding us back from realizing our full potential. These unseen weights shape our thoughts, actions, and interactions, hindering personal growth and robbing us of inner peace. The first step toward freedom is recognizing the specific ways these burdens influence our lives. They might appear as self-doubt, preventing someone from seizing opportunities or believing in their own abilities. They might appear as unspoken frustrations, straining relationships, or clouding our sense of purpose. Understanding these emotions means seeing them clearly and acknowledging their grip on our mindset and daily lives.

There's power in understanding the difference between internal and external sources of emotional burdens. Internal struggles often stem from within, like when you criticize yourself for not achieving your goals as quickly as you think you should, even though you've made significant progress. You may hold on to past mistakes, regret decisions you've made, and find yourself trapped in a cycle of negative self-talk that undermines your confidence.

On the other hand, external pressures arise from outside forces. You might feel overwhelmed by societal expectations to meet certain standards of success, whether it's in your career, appearance, or lifestyle, even though these ideals don't align with your true desires. Similarly, family expectations can weigh heavily, with pressure to follow a particular career path or make certain life choices, even when they don't resonate with your personal values. Both internal and external burdens can feel suffocating, but they require different approaches—internal struggles call for self-compassion and reframing, while external pressures require setting boundaries and aligning with your own values.

The key to alleviating these burdens lies in acknowledgment. Confronting the thoughts and emotions that weigh us down is no easy task, but it is the vital first step toward healing. Genuine introspection enables us to identify our burdens, comprehend their origins, and recognize their effects. This awareness is enlightening—it converts emotional weight into an opportunity for change and personal growth.

Reflection is a transformative tool on this journey. Taking time to sit with your feelings—through journaling or quiet contemplation—can bring hidden emotions to light. Writing, for example, offers a safe space to explore recurring thoughts, uncovering patterns that reveal the true source of your struggles. Questions like "What am I holding on to?" or "Whose approval matters most to me?" can be eye-opening, guiding you toward clarity and release.

Establishing a regular practice of self-reflection deepens this process. Whether it's a few moments each morning or a weekly check-in, dedicating time to explore what feels heavy—and why—can be extremely liberating. Reflection reveals the burdens we carry and helps us envision a lighter, freer future.

Recognizing and addressing emotional burdens is a courageous act that sets the stage for healing and resilience. By naming our fears, inse-curities, and pressures, we strip them of their power. As researchers like Kohrt and colleagues (2020) highlight, healing begins with empathy and self-awareness—skills that grow as we confront what holds us back. Under-standing and integrating our emotions allows us to change our burdens into stepping stones, using them to build strength, clarity, and peace. The journey may be challenging, but it is worthwhile. Confronting each burden brings you closer to the freedom to grow, thrive, and embrace your fullest self.

HOW STRESS PHYSICALLY CHANGES YOUR BRAIN

Stress is not just a mental or emotional experience—it causes physical changes in the brain that can affect memory, decision-making, emotional regulation, and overall cognitive function. While short-term stress can be beneficial by enhancing focus and alertness, chronic stress has lasting negative effects on brain structure and function. The main culprit behind these changes is cortisol, the body's primary stress hormone. When stress becomes prolonged, excessive cortisol exposure can lead to shrinkage in key brain regions, disrupted neural connections, and imbalances in brain chemistry.

Shrinking of the Prefrontal Cortex: Harder Decision-Making and More Emotional Reactions

The prefrontal cortex is a part of the brain that helps with decision-making, self-control, and managing emotions. When stress is constant, this part of the brain shrinks, making it harder to focus, control impulses, and think through problems logically. This can lead to feeling overwhelmed, reacting emotionally to minor issues, or making quick decisions that might not be the best. Over time, it can affect schoolwork, relationships, and confidence in handling challenges (Arnsten et al., 2012).

Overactive Amygdala: Increased Anxiety and Fear

The amygdala is like the brain's alarm system—it detects threats and triggers fear responses. When stress is ongoing, the amygdala grows larger and becomes more sensitive, making you feel more anxious, jumpy, or on edge, even when there's no real danger. This can lead to constant worrying, difficulty relaxing, and even panic attacks. The more stress continues, the harder it becomes to calm down, which can impact sleep, focus, and mood.

Damage to the Hippocampus: Memory Problems and Trouble Learning

The hippocampus is the brain's memory center, helping you remember facts, events, and experiences. Chronic stress weakens this part of the brain, making it harder to remember things, learn new information, or recall details for exams. It's why people under stress often feel forgetful or mentally exhausted. Over time, this damage can also increase the risk of conditions like depression and post-traumatic stress disorder (*5 Ways Stress Can Impact Your Memory*, n.d.).

Imbalanced Brain Chemistry:
Mood Swings and Lack of Motivation

Stress affects the balance of brain chemicals like dopamine, serotonin, and norepinephrine, which control mood, motivation, and energy levels. When these chemicals are disrupted, it can lead to feeling down, irritability, or a lack of drive to do things you normally enjoy. This is one reason why stress and burnout often lead to feelings of hopelessness or emotional exhaustion (Raypole, 2022).

Weaker Brain Connections:
Less Creativity and Problem-Solving Ability

Neurons in the brain communicate through connections called synapses. Long-term stress weakens these connections, making it harder for different parts of the brain to work together. This can lead to trouble adapting to new situations, struggling to come up with solutions to problems, and feeling stuck in negative thought patterns. Over time, stress can cause you to feel less flexible in your thinking, limiting creativity and problem-solving skills (McEwen, 2017).

Inflammation in the Brain:
Higher Risk of Mental Health Issues

Chronic stress increases inflammation in the brain, which has been linked to mental health conditions like anxiety, depression, and even long-term brain diseases. The more the brain stays in a stressed state, the harder it is to regulate emotions and stay mentally healthy (McEwen, 2017).

Disrupted Sleep and Weaker Immune System

The hypothalamic-pituitary-adrenal axis controls how the body reacts to stress. When it stays overactive, cortisol levels remain high, making it difficult to sleep, leaving you constantly tired, and weakening the immune system. This means stress can not only make you feel mentally exhausted but can also make you physically sick more often (*How the Outdoors Can Improve Your Mood*, 2024).

Stress is a part of life, but learning how to manage it can prevent these negative effects on the brain. Taking breaks, getting enough sleep, exercising, and talking to someone about your worries can all help keep stress from taking control. Your brain is always changing, and the good news is that positive habits can help it heal and stay strong.

RECOGNIZING THE IMPACT ON MENTAL HEALTH

Emotional burdens, though often unseen, can significantly impact our mental health and overall well-being, hindering personal growth and peace. These burdens, whether from stress, guilt, or unresolved conflicts, create a cycle of anxiety and physical symptoms, such as fatigue and irritability. Left unaddressed, they can lead to long-term mental health issues and unhealthy coping behaviors. However, by recognizing these struggles and prioritizing emotional intelligence, support, and self-care, individuals can break the cycle and encourage resilience, clarity, and improved relationships, ultimately leading to a more balanced and fulfilling life.

A consequence of unaddressed emotional burdens is the rise in stress and anxiety. While stress is a natural response to life's demands, it becomes problematic when it persists over time. The connection between emotional burdens and stress is significant; unresolved emotions can create a cycle where stress feeds anxiety, and anxiety exacerbates the feelings tied to those burdens. When this happens, individuals may experience physiological changes, such as increased heart rate and cortisol levels, which might increase the risk of cardiovascular issues (Peterson, 2023). Long-term stress not only harms physical health but also leads to cognitive impairments such as memory loss and decreased decision-making ability. This interrelation highlights the importance of recognizing and managing emotional burdens early on.

Recognizing the symptoms that signal a struggle with emotional burdens is essential. Individuals facing these challenges might find themselves withdrawing socially, a common response when dealing with overwhelming emotions. Withdrawal can manifest as avoiding social situations, reducing interactions with friends and family, or isolating oneself for extended periods.

Another symptom is irritability, where minor inconveniences trigger disproportionate reactions. Emotional burdens can lead to heightened sensitivity, resulting in frequent bouts of anger or frustration without apparent cause. Fatigue is also a significant indicator; it's more than just feeling tired. Emotional fatigue saps one's energy and motivation, making even simple tasks seem daunting. Recognizing symptoms like withdrawal, irritability, and fatigue makes it easier to identify the underlying emotional issues that require attention.

Emotional burdens, left unaddressed, can lead to severe long-term mental health issues, such as chronic anxiety, depression, and other mood disorders. Prolonged exposure to unresolved stress increases allostatic load, the "wear and tear" on the body caused by fluctuations in hormones (Aquin et al., 2017). This added stress heightens the risk of developing physical health conditions, which in turn complicates mental health struggles. Furthermore, neglecting emotional well-being can encourage maladaptive behaviors, such as substance abuse or poor eating habits, as temporary escapes. While these behaviors may offer brief relief, they ultimately prevent the development of healthy coping mechanisms and worsen mental health over time (Peterson, 2023).

Proactively engaging with your emotions is important in preventing these long-term consequences. Emotional intelligence plays a significant role here, allowing you to understand and manage your feelings effectively. Encouraging dialogue about what you're feeling, whether through professional therapy or supportive conversations with loved ones, fosters an environment where you feel safe expressing yourself. Techniques like mindfulness and meditation can help you connect with your emotions, providing clarity and perspective. Actively addressing emotional burdens helps you equip yourself with tools to manage stressors more effectively, reducing their impact on your mental health.

Prioritizing mental health is paramount in achieving emotional wholeness and clarity. Mental health should be viewed with the same importance as physical health, as they are closely intertwined. An effective mental health strategy includes regular self-evaluation to prevent unresolved feelings from building up inside. Incorporating self-care practices, such as engaging in hobbies and maintaining a balanced diet, is essential for promoting overall well-being. Structuring time for relaxation and reflection can help prevent feeling overwhelmed, and emphasizing the importance of rest and leisure activities promotes a balanced lifestyle. Concentrating on mental health lays a solid foundation for enhanced emotional strength, empowering individuals to face life's obstacles with greater confidence.

Taking care of emotional health leads to clearer thinking and stronger relationships. When we prioritize mental health, communication improves, making it easier to express our needs and feelings without avoiding or becoming defensive. Healthy relationships are built on openness and understanding, which are supported by good mental health habits. Greater mental clarity also improves decision-making, helping us to make choices that align with our values and goals, free from the influence of unresolved emotional issues.

CONNECTION BETWEEN PAST EXPERIENCES AND CURRENT DISTRESS

Past experiences, especially trauma, leave lasting imprints that shape our current emotional burdens and reactions. Understanding how these unresolved events affect us can be complex but enlightening, as they influence how we respond to new situations and relationships.

Trauma fundamentally shakes our sense of security and stability, forming neural pathways that are more reactive to stress and negative experiences. This change can make it challenging to be fully present, as unresolved emotions and memories from the past may influence current perceptions and interactions. As a result, individuals may become trapped in a cycle where their past continues to affect them, unknowingly hindering their ability to embrace growth and change (Lee, n.d.).

Consider Emily, who grew up in a home where emotional neglect and uncertainty were constant. As she entered adulthood, she struggled with feelings of inadequacy and had difficulty forming meaningful connections. It wasn't until she began examining her past and recognizing the impact these early experiences had on her sense of self-worth that she started her healing journey. Through therapy and personal growth practices, Emily was able to transform the weight of her past into a source of empowerment, showing resilience and strength by embracing her story and choosing to heal.

Emily's story reflects the power of resilience in overcoming the struggles tied to past wounds. It serves as a reminder that while the past may influence who we are, it does not have to define us. We all have the potential to grow, but it requires introspection and the willingness to confront painful memories in order to move forward.

A practical approach to understanding the impact of one's past is to engage in reflective practices such as journaling. Journaling serves as a tool for self-discovery, offering a safe space to explore thoughts and emotions related to past experiences. Writing things down allows individuals to gain insight into how past events have shaped their mindset and behaviors. Reflective writing promotes honesty and vulnerability, helping one process emotions and gradually let go of the grip that past experiences may have on them.

Embracing forgiveness is crucial for letting go of past grievances. It serves as an impactful gesture, benefiting not only others but, more importantly, oneself. Forgiveness helps us let go of resentment and emotional baggage, liberating us from holding on to negativity. It's about developing empathy, both toward those who may have wronged us and toward ourselves. Embracing forgiveness requires courage and a shift in perspective, focusing on personal healing instead of dwelling on past grievances.

Imagine someone lugging around a heavy backpack filled with rocks everywhere they go. Each step becomes increasingly laborious, and the weight eventually takes a toll on their spirit and well-being. This metaphor captures what life feels like when we hold on to grudges and resentments—it is exhausting and limiting. Forgiveness allows us to unload these rocks, lightening the load and paving the way for a more fulfilling life.

Teenagers and young adults need to learn about the power of forgiveness, as it can be a life-changing experience. It helps build emotional intelligence, encouraging healthier approaches to challenges and relationships. Parents, guardians, and educators also play an integral role in supporting youths by encouraging these practices and creating environments conducive to emotional growth and resilience.

To initiate the forgiving process, individuals can practice self-compassion by acknowledging their pain without judgment. This internal acknowledgment opens a space for empathetic reflection, which is fundamental for letting go of past hurts. It's not about excusing harmful actions but regaining control over one's emotional landscape and refusing to let painful past events dictate the present or future.

Integrating mindfulness practices into daily routines can complement reflective practices. These strategies enhance self-awareness by grounding individuals in the present moment and reducing the mental noise created by past burdens. Mindfulness teaches people to observe their emotions without getting swept away by them, which is particularly helpful when dealing with emotional wounds from the past.

Building supportive networks is also essential for healing. Sharing your journey with trusted friends, family, or support groups creates a foundation of encouragement and strength. Connecting with those who truly understand and empathize creates a safe space where you can freely express emotions and begin the process of forgiveness. Professional counseling offers personalized guidance, equipping you with the tools and strategies needed to navigate the complex path of emotional recovery with confidence and resilience.

STRATEGIES FOR ACKNOWLEDGMENT AND ACCEPTANCE

Understanding Emotional Burdens

Understanding and accepting emotional burdens is essential for anyone seeking personal growth and inner peace. One of the first steps in this journey is acknowledgment, a powerful tool that paves the way for change. Recognizing the existence of these burdens allows individuals to confront and work through them rather than letting them linger unaddressed. Acknowledgment is about observing one's feelings without judgment, which can offer clarity and pave the way forward.

The Power of Acknowledgment

The power of acknowledgment lies in its ability to shift one's perspective. Naming the emotional weights we carry allows us to remove the ambiguity and fear surrounding those feelings. This is the first step toward emotional change, as it offers a clear understanding of what requires attention. Simply identifying each emotional burden helps to untangle complex emotions and provides a foundation for deeper reflection and healing.

The Importance of Acceptance

Once we acknowledge our burdens, the next important step is acceptance, which often requires a kind and compassionate approach toward oneself. Techniques like self-compassion and affirmations are invaluable here. Self-compassion involves treating ourselves with the same understanding and kindness we would offer a friend. It encourages forgiveness and patience during times of struggle, helping us to accept our imperfections and mistakes as part of the human experience.

The Role of Affirmations

Affirmations are positive statements that remind us of our intrinsic worth and capacity for growth. Regularly repeating affirmations such as "I am worthy of love and acceptance" or "I embrace my emotions as part of my journey" helps rewire negative thought patterns. These practices foster a nurturing internal environment where acceptance can flourish, reducing resistance and promoting emotional well-being.

Introspective Activities for Healing

Quiet activities dedicated to introspection, such as art therapy or nature walks, offer individuals a safe space for self-reflection and emotional healing. Art therapy, for example, allows individuals to express complex emotions through creative outlets such as drawing, painting, or sculpting. This non-verbal form of expression can help people connect with their inner selves, providing clarity and relief from emotional burdens. For instance, someone dealing with grief might find solace in painting abstract images that represent their sorrow, eventually channeling their emotions into something tangible. Over time, this process can facilitate healing by externalizing feelings that are difficult to articulate.

The Benefits of Nature Walks

Nature walks also serve as an excellent method for introspection and emotional clarity. The peaceful environment of a forest, park, or beach offers a soothing backdrop for quiet reflection. Walking among the trees or by the water can encourage mindfulness, as the natural world invites individuals to be fully present in the moment. For example, a person feeling overwhelmed by stress might take a walk through a nearby park, focusing on the sounds of the birds or the rustling of leaves. As they immerse themselves in nature, the act of walking combined with the calming influence of the surroundings can help release tension and bring a sense of balance.

The Path to Healing

Carrying emotional burdens is a natural part of life, but these weights don't have to define who we are or limit what we can achieve. Recognizing what we carry, understanding its source, and handling it with care opens the door to healing. The process of letting go allows for the reclamation of energy, the strengthening of relationships, and the cultivation of inner peace, paving the way for a more satisfying and genuine life.

The Role of Self-Awareness

Self-awareness serves as an invaluable partner on this path, revealing the hidden influences that shape our actions and decisions. Aligning our choices with our true values and recognizing what truly matters leads to a greater sense of freedom and purpose. Reflection, mindfulness, and building supportive relationships serve as essential resources to guide this path, turning emotional burdens into stepping stones for growth and resilience.

As we prepare to explore Chapter 2, "The Art of Letting Go," we will take a fundamental step toward shedding the weight of our past. Embracing this art allows us to let go of what no longer serves us while creating room for new experiences, perspectives, and opportunities. The path forward will reveal important practices that enable us to release limiting beliefs and adopt a more rewarding life, encouraging us to discover the beauty and freedom found in genuinely letting go.

KEY TAKEAWAYS

- Emotional burdens such as guilt, anxiety, and societal pressures can profoundly affect our lives and obstruct personal development.

- Acknowledging and understanding these burdens is essential for healing and self-growth, as they influence our thoughts and relationships.

- Emotional burdens can arise from internal factors like self-criticism or external ones like family expectations and societal pressures, each requiring a different approach for resolution.

- Practices like self-reflection, mindfulness, and open self-dialogue can help identify and manage these emotional burdens, promoting growth and resilience.

- Chronic stress can disrupt brain function, impairing memory, decision-making, and emotional regulation, which exacerbates the impact of emotional burdens on mental health.

- Focusing on mental well-being through self-awareness, emotional intelligence, and strong, supportive relationships can enhance overall health and help release the hold of past influences.

CHAPTER 2

The Art of Letting Go

Emotional freedom begins with the courage
to release old wounds and embrace
the strength of new possibilities.

Releasing our past burdens is a powerful practice that allows us to let go of old wounds and liberate ourselves from unhelpful habits. It's a journey toward emotional freedom, where unburdening ourselves opens the door to healing and growth. Though the concept may sound simple, its impact can be life-changing. Letting go requires courage, intentional action, and moments of deep reflection—essential steps toward reclaiming peace and discovering the strength within.

This chapter explores practical and meaningful ways to embrace this process. Mindful journaling creates a judgment-free space for processing emotions, while visualization techniques empower the mind to imagine and accept positive change. Connecting with nature provides grounding and serenity, reminding us of life's beauty beyond our personal struggles. Practices like yoga and other mindful movements help release both physical and emotional tension, nurturing a sense of balance and inner calm. Together, these techniques form a powerful toolkit for change, offering a path toward resilience, self-awareness, and lasting emotional freedom. Through these practices, you will uncover new possibilities for healing and learn to embrace the art of letting go with grace and purpose.

MINDFULNESS EXERCISES FOR LETTING GO

Mindfulness exercises are effective tools for helping you release emotional burdens and enhancing your self-connection. This section explores techniques that promote emotional healing and self-discovery, including mindful journaling, visualization, nature immersion, and mindful movement. Each method encourages you to embrace your feelings, reflect on your experiences, and cultivate inner peace.

Mindful Journaling

This practice promotes emotional freedom by helping you release past pain. It can provide you with a private space for reflection, allowing for deeper self-awareness and emotional clarity.

HOW TO PRACTICE

1. Set aside quiet time for writing, free from distractions.
2. Begin by focusing on your breath to center yourself.
3. Write freely about your thoughts, feelings, and experiences without judgment.
4. Reflect on any patterns or emotions that arise during the process.
5. Allow yourself to express even the rawest, unspoken feelings on paper.
6. Conclude by rereading your writing and acknowledging any insights gained.

Mindful journaling acts as a tool for your emotional release and self-discovery. Establishing a space for introspection enables you to analyze your thoughts and feelings objectively, leading to enhanced self-awareness and insight.

What physical feelings do I go through when I am stressed or overwhelmed?

_____

_____

_____

_____

_____

_____

When I think about my current mental health, what feelings come up first? For example:

- I feel overwhelmed.
- I feel anxious about the future.
- I feel a sense of emptiness.
- I feel frustrated with myself.
- I feel sad and alone.
- I feel hopeless.
- I feel pressured to stay positive.

_____

_____

_____

_____

What small steps can I take today to relieve stress and nurture my mental well-being?

_____

_____

_____

_____

_____

_____

_____

_____

Visualization Techniques

Visualization techniques are another tool for encouraging emotional release and healing. These methods involve creating mental imagery that aligns with your desired outcomes or feelings. Visualizing a serene place or a comforting scenario allows you to mentally step away from stressors and find your inner peace. This practice acts as a rehearsal for your positive change, helping your mind focus on possibilities rather than limitations.

HOW TO PRACTICE

1. Imagine yourself in a situation where you've been holding on to anger or resentment toward someone.
2. Close your eyes and take several deep, calming breaths.
3. Picture the anger as a dark, heavy cloud surrounding your chest, its weight pressing on you.
4. Visualize yourself slowly releasing the cloud.
5. Watch the cloud dissolve as you exhale, feeling the tension in your body ease with every breath.
6. As the cloud disappears, imagine a warm, soothing light filling the space where the anger once was.
7. Allow this light to bring peace and clarity.
8. Consider combining this mental exercise with deep breathing or meditation to reinforce a sense of calm and control.

Getting Out Into Nature

Nature immersion is a powerful mindfulness practice that promotes letting go and encourages a sense of connectedness and tranquility. Engaging with natural environments—such as walking barefoot on the grass, listening to birds, or feeling the breeze—anchors you in the present moment and enhances your overall well-being.

HOW TO PRACTICE

1. Take a walk in a park, forest, or on a beach.
2. Feel the earth beneath your feet, listen to the sounds of nature, and observe your surroundings.
3. Let go of distractions and immerse yourself in the tranquility of the natural world.
4. Breathe deeply and notice how nature helps ground you in the moment.

Engaging with nature also encourages a broader perspective. Being amid trees or near water can remind one of life's vastness, reducing the perceived importance of personal grievances. According to Susan Albers, PsyD, a psychologist at the Cleveland Clinic, spending 15 minutes a day outside can lower cortisol levels and improve your overall mood (*How the Outdoors Can Improve Your Mood*, 2024).

Mindful Movement

Incorporating mindful movements such as yoga into your daily routine can significantly facilitate emotional release. Yoga intertwines physical poses with breath awareness, promoting a state of presence during your practice. As you release tension through targeted stretching and strengthening, your emotional burdens begin to fade away. Numerous yoga practices exist to effectively alleviate stress and tension, which you will explore further in Chapter 7.

The benefits of mindful movement extend beyond the physical realm. Practicing yoga regularly can help you build resilience against stress and enhance your self-awareness. It teaches you to accept your body's abilities and limits, promoting self-compassion and patience. Focusing on breath and sensation helps you tune into your body, making it easier to recognize and address stored emotional tensions.

Each of these mindfulness techniques presents distinct benefits, and incorporating one or all into your daily life can lead to emotional healing. By incorporating these practices into your daily life, you can establish a comprehensive strategy for emotional well-being, promoting greater self-awareness and clarity.

COGNITIVE BEHAVIORAL STRATEGIES

In the journey to emotional freedom, recognizing and changing unproductive thought patterns is a pivotal step. Understanding how our minds can trap us in cycles of negativity allows us to break free from them. This section explores cognitive behavioral techniques designed to challenge and change those unproductive thoughts, opening the door to a more positive mindset.

Recognizing negative thoughts is a key step toward meaningful change. These thoughts often disguise themselves as truths, quietly shaping how we see ourselves and the world. Paying close attention to your inner dialogue helps you identify and understand the triggers behind harmful self-talk. For example, if you often think *I'm not good enough*, learning to spot that pattern is essential. Writing these thoughts down in a journal can be incredibly helpful—it brings awareness and gives you a way to spot recurring themes over time. Recognizing your thoughts impartially allows them to flow freely without exerting control over you, creating a foundation for a more positive mindset.

Once negative thoughts are identified, cognitive restructuring becomes an effective tool in reframing them. This technique involves critically assessing and altering distorted thinking patterns to ensure a healthier perspective. Consider the thought, *I always fail*. Cognitive restructuring encourages breaking down such absolutes by exploring evidence that counters them. Did you succeed in recent tasks? Have there been instances when you overcame challenges? Consciously focusing on positives helps diminish the overwhelming power of negativity. Exercises such as thought records, where situations, emotions, automatic thoughts, and rational responses are logged, provide tangible proof of progress. Over time, adopting a balanced view helps diminish the influence of anxiety and depression, encouraging long-term shifts in mindset.

Behavioral activation complements cognitive efforts by urging engagement in fulfilling activities that enhance mood and routine. Sometimes, negativity arises from both thought and a lack of action or disconnection. Engaging in activities known to bring joy or satisfaction—whether it's taking a walk, painting, or spending time with friends—helps disrupt negative spirals. This approach is rooted in action rather than introspection, promoting a break from unhealthy patterns through active participation in life. Research by Craft and Perna (2004) highlights that physical activity helps to relieve depressive feelings. Scheduling regular time for hobbies and interests aids in constructing a more joyful and predictable routine, which is fundamental to maintaining mental wellness.

Setting boundaries plays an important role in preserving personal well-being and encouraging empowerment. Learning when and how to say no is an act of self-respect and protection against unwanted stress and obligations. Boundaries create a clear line between one's needs and external demands, reducing the likelihood of burnout and resentment. When a young adult decides to prioritize their studies over social events, asserting that boundary helps reinforce their commitment to personal growth. Empowerment comes from honoring oneself, which in turn cultivates healthier connections with others.

To illustrate, consider a teenager overwhelmed by peer pressure to conform to certain pressures at school. Identifying the trigger—the fear of missing out—and consciously setting a boundary around it empowers individuals to regain control over their decisions. Let's explore this a bit more in the next section.

Boundaries to Combat Common High School Peer Pressures

High school is often a time when teens feel immense pressure to conform to the expectations of their peers. Setting clear boundaries can help combat these pressures and foster self-confidence, authenticity, and resilience. Below are a few peer pressures and the boundaries that can help teens manage them effectively.

FASHION TRENDS

Teens often feel the need to follow the latest fashion trends or wear specific brands to fit in with popular groups. While it's natural to want to belong, this pressure can lead to overspending or compromising personal style.

- **Boundary:** "I will wear clothes that make me feel comfortable and confident, regardless of trends."
- **Action:** Embrace your individuality by developing a personal style and resisting the urge to follow every trend.

SOCIAL MEDIA IMAGE

Maintaining a curated social media presence can create a constant need for validation and approval. Teens may feel pressured to post frequently, participate in trends, or portray a perfect life.

- **Boundary:** "I won't post or engage in social media just to seek approval from others."
- **Action:** Limit screen time and focus on sharing content that aligns with your values rather than chasing likes or trends.

ATTENDING PARTIES

Many teens feel compelled to attend parties, even if they are uncomfortable or uninterested, simply to avoid being labeled as "uncool." This can lead to compromising personal values or engaging in risky behaviors.

- **Boundary:** "I will only attend social events that I genuinely want to be part of and feel safe attending."
- **Action:** Politely decline invitations that don't align with your comfort level, and suggest other ways to connect with friends.

ROMANTIC RELATIONSHIPS

The pressure to have a boyfriend or girlfriend can be intense, as it is often seen as a status symbol among peers. Teens may feel rushed into relationships they are not ready for or genuinely interested in.

- **Boundary:** "I won't feel pressured to be in a relationship just because others expect it."

- **Action:** Focus on building meaningful friendships and developing self-confidence before pursuing romantic relationships.

SUBSTANCE USE

Experimenting with alcohol, vaping, or drugs is a common pressure teenagers face in high school. Teens may feel compelled to participate to avoid being judged or excluded.

- **Boundary:** "I will not use substances like alcohol, vaping, or drugs, even if others are doing so."
- **Action:** Practice saying "no" firmly and confidently, and create an exit plan for situations where pressure arises.

BODY IMAGE STANDARDS

Unrealistic beauty standards and peer-driven fitness expectations can lead to harmful comparisons and unhealthy habits. Teens often feel the need to look a certain way to fit in.

- **Boundary:** "I won't compare my body to others or engage in unhealthy habits to meet unrealistic standards."
- **Action:** Prioritize health and self-acceptance, and surround yourself with supportive people who value you for who you are.

EXTRACURRICULAR PARTICIPATION

Teens may feel obligated to join certain clubs or sports teams for social status, even if they have no genuine interest in the activities themselves.

- **Boundary:** "I will only join activities that genuinely interest me and align with my goals."
- **Action:** Explore hobbies and extracurriculars that bring joy and fulfillment, regardless of their popularity.

FRIEND GROUP LOYALTY

Toxic friendships can trap teens into staying in unhealthy relationships out of fear of social isolation. This can hinder personal growth and self-esteem.

- **Boundary:** "I will distance myself from toxic friendships and invest in relationships that uplift me."
- **Action:** Choose friends who respect your boundaries and encourage your authenticity.

MUSIC AND POP CULTURE PREFERENCES

Teens often feel pressured to like specific music, shows, or influencers to fit in with their peer group. This can suppress their true preferences and individuality.

- **Boundary:** "I will enjoy the music and shows I like, even if they're not popular among my peers."
- **Action:** Share your interests confidently and seek out others who share similar tastes.

CLASSROOM BEHAVIOR

Peer pressure in the classroom can lead to adopting disruptive or disengaged behaviors to avoid being seen as a "teacher's pet" or "nerd."

- **Boundary:** "I will stay true to my learning goals and avoid mimicking behavior that disrupts my education."
- **Action:** Focus on your academic success and build connections with peers who share your commitment to learning.

Establishing boundaries in key areas enables teenagers to withstand social pressures and foster healthier connections, enhancing their self-confidence and overall well-being. These limits empower them to make decisions that reflect their principles, cultivating a more robust sense of identity.

CREATING RITUALS FOR RELEASE

Personal rituals have a way of helping us heal, offering powerful tools for letting go of emotional pain and old patterns that no longer serve us. They bring a sense of stability and purpose when life feels overwhelming. More than just routines, these rituals become personal and meaningful acts of intention, helping us move forward with mindfulness and a renewed sense of peace.

One prominent ritual is that of forgiveness, a practice that cultivates healing from past wounds. Forgiveness does not merely mean forgetting or dismissing grievances but rather confronting them with the compassion to release their hold on us. This act can be seen as a liberating gesture, where we choose to no longer be bound by the chains of resentment and hurt. Creating a personal ritual of forgiveness opens the door to emotional freedom, allowing life's pain to evolve into lessons of strength and resilience.

Consider crafting a simple yet effective forgiveness ritual: writing letters expressing your feelings without holding back to those who have wronged you. However, these letters are not meant for delivery; instead, they're destined for a symbolic release through burning. As the paper turns to ash, visualize the anger and pain dissipating with the smoke, leaving behind a lighter heart. This practice helps articulate emotions powerfully, providing closure and clearing the path for new beginnings (Elise, 2019).

Healing ceremonies also play a vital role in marking significant transitions, signifying the movement from familiar habits to renewed commitments. Such ceremonies can be tailored to suit individual or group settings, encouraging a shared sense of purpose and accountability. Through activities like lighting candles, chanting affirmations, or creating a vision board, participants reinforce their dedication to change. These ceremonies emphasize the significance of honoring each step toward personal growth, strengthening our resolve to shed what no longer serves us.

Symbolic acts, like letter burning, extend beyond written words. They encompass any tangible actions that represent the release of burdens. Planting a seed is another powerful symbolic act—a metaphor for turning grief or loss into hope and renewal. As you plant the seed, picture your painful memories being turned into nurturing soil that brings new life. With time, this small act blossoms into a reminder that change is possible, nurturing both the heart and the spirit. Such symbolic gestures create safe spaces for emotional exploration, promoting courage and introspection.

Gratitude rituals also stand out as essential practices that redirect focus toward appreciation and positivity. In moments of distress, it's easy to lose sight of what remains good and fulfilling. Gratitude rituals counterbalance this tendency by encouraging a shift in perspective. Start a daily gratitude journal where you write down things—big or small—that bring joy and encouragement. This simple habit encourages an environment of positivity, which in turn nurtures emotional well-being and resilience over time (Walsh, 2015).

Here are three gratitude journaling prompts to get you started:

What is one thing I'm grateful for today, and why does it matter to me?

_____

_____

_____

_____

_____

_____

_____

Whom do I currently feel supported by, and in what specific ways can I express my gratitude to them?

What is something about myself that I'm thankful for, whether it's a strength, talent, or quality?

_____

_____

_____

_____

_____

_____

_____

_____

_____

_____

_____

_____

_____

The science behind these rituals highlights their impact on our brain's functioning. Our brains, naturally geared toward familiarity, often resist change due to fear of the unknown (Elise, 2019). Engaging in purposeful rituals trains our minds to associate these changes with safety and comfort, making the transition smoother. This intentionality empowers us to break free from habitual constraints, forging paths toward healthier behaviors and mindsets. Rituals anchor our intentions, directing focus and energy toward constructive goals.

For instance, adolescents and young adults grappling with emotional challenges may find solace in customized rituals that resonate with their struggles. Whether it's crafting vision boards that depict future aspirations or hosting communal ceremonies with friends, practicing these simple exercises demonstrates the shift from a passive experience to active participation in one's healing journey. The autonomy and creativity involved in designing personal rituals encourage empowerment, which is crucial for building self-awareness and emotional intelligence.

Personal rituals are powerful practices that facilitate healing, promote growth, and establish stability in the face of life's difficulties. Participating in acts of forgiveness, showing appreciation, or undertaking significant gestures helps us lighten our emotional burdens, build resilience, and achieve clearer insights.

BUILDING A SUPPORT SYSTEM

Personal growth and emotional healing can feel overwhelming, especially for teens and young adults facing emotional challenges. But having a supportive community around you can make all the difference. Whether it's friends, family, or mentors, positive relationships offer stability and reassurance, reminding you that you're not alone in your journey. These connections help build self-esteem and a healthier outlook on life. Open communication is key—it creates a space where you can be vulnerable without fear of judgment, strengthening your emotional resilience. Support groups also offer a sense of belonging, where shared experiences help ease feelings of isolation and encourage healing. And for deeper challenges, professional counseling can provide the tools and guidance needed to work through tough emotions and develop healthier coping strategies. With the right support, growth and healing are always possible.

Identifying Supportive Figures

One of the most important steps in emotional healing is recognizing the supportive individuals in your life. Friends, family, and mentors can significantly contribute to promoting emotional well-being and personal development. These figures serve as anchors during difficult times, offering stability and helping boost self-esteem. Their encouragement reminds you that you are not alone, making it easier to face challenges with a positive outlook.

The Power of Open Communication

Open communication helps to create a safe space for emotional expression. In relationships built on trust, individuals can freely share their thoughts and feelings without fear of judgment. This openness ensures mutual understanding, which deepens connections and builds emotional resilience. Verbalizing your emotions also aids in processing them, leading to emotional clarity and relief. Discussing obstacles candidly can significantly facilitate emotional recovery.

The Role of Support Groups

Support groups offer a valuable platform for shared experiences and mutual understanding. These groups bring together people who are experiencing similar struggles, creating a sense of belonging and helping individuals realize they are not alone. As noted by the Mayo Clinic Staff (2025), support groups encourage camaraderie, allowing participants to share coping strategies and personal insights, which can illuminate paths toward healing. This collective environment empowers individuals with new perspectives and encourages emotional growth.

Seeking Professional Help

When facing deeper personal issues, professional therapy or counseling offers valuable guidance to navigate tough emotions. Therapists are trained to help individuals explore underlying challenges and provide tools and techniques to process emotions and develop healthier coping strategies. Support is vital when addressing entrenched thought patterns and behaviors. Therapy establishes a safe framework for self-reflection, fostering significant personal development and emotional healing.

Personal growth and emotional healing thrive through collective support. Creating a community of supportive people, encouraging open conversations, participating in support groups, and seeking professional advice are essential for building a solid foundation of emotional well-being. These resources provide assurance and strength, enabling you to manage your feelings, develop resilience, and embrace healthier coping strategies. With the right support, healing becomes achievable, and personal growth transforms into an ongoing, enriching journey.

Letting go is a powerful practice that allows us to release the hold of past pain and let go of patterns that no longer support our growth. It is a journey toward emotional freedom, where unburdening ourselves clears the way for healing and progress. Although the concept appears simple, its effect can be significant. Letting go takes courage, intentional action, and deep reflection—key steps toward regaining peace and discovering inner strength.

As we move on to the next chapter, we will explore building emotional resilience—a vital component of the healing process. Releasing past burdens paves the way for developing the emotional fortitude necessary to confront challenges with poise and assurance. We will explore how cultivating resilience enables us to adapt, recover, and emerge stronger from life's inevitable challenges. Through the practices outlined in this chapter, we will learn how to nurture our minds and become resilient individuals.

KEY TAKEAWAYS

- Letting go of past burdens promotes emotional freedom, enabling individuals to heal and grow by releasing old wounds and unhelpful behaviors.

- Practices like journaling, visualization, spending time in nature, and mindful movement support emotional healing and self-discovery.

- Journaling mindfully helps encourage clarity and self-awareness, while visualization techniques assist in mentally letting go of negative emotions.

- Engaging with nature boosts well-being by offering tranquility and grounding, which can reduce stress and provide valuable perspective.

- Cognitive behavioral techniques empower individuals to challenge unhelpful thought patterns and build resilience through recognition and reframing.

- Building a supportive community through open communication, support groups, and professional counseling is essential for personal growth and emotional healing.

CHAPTER 3

Building Emotional Resilience

Resilience isn't merely about enduring challenges; it's about growing through adversity and coming out stronger than before.

Developing emotional resilience is essential for individuals as they face the various challenges that arise during different phases of life. Emotional resilience is the ability to cope with adversity, recover from setbacks, and keep moving forward with strength. Think of it as having an emotional toolbox that helps manage stress, bounce back from difficulties, and maintain mental well-being through life's unpredictable moments. In today's fast-paced world, developing this resilience is more essential than ever. It allows individuals not only to endure tough times but also to grow and thrive through them.

UNDERSTANDING RESILIENCE AND ITS BENEFITS

Resilience is vital for navigating life's challenges. It's often defined as the ability to adapt when faced with adversity, trauma, or stress (Hurley, 2024). Resilience is more than just bouncing back; it's about using the insights gained from these experiences to move forward with greater strength and understanding. Recognizing how resilience contributes to personal growth and emotional stability helps us focus on developing the traits that enable us to handle life's difficulties more effectively.

The Benefits Of Resilience

The benefits of resilience extend beyond merely surviving difficult times. Individuals who cultivate resilience tend to exhibit improved emotional regulation, which enables them to handle stress more effectively. Emotional regulation enables individuals to process their feelings in healthy ways instead of being overwhelmed by them. This enables them to build stronger connections with peers, mentors, and family through clearer and more compassionate communication.

Enhanced coping skills are another advantage of resilience. These skills equip individuals with the tools to face new challenges head-on. Resilient individuals tackle challenges head-on by employing effective problem-solving techniques and reaching out for support when needed. This proactive approach encourages them to view challenges not as insurmountable problems but as opportunities for learning and growth.

Real-world examples vividly illustrate the deep impact resilience can have on our lives. Consider the experience of someone who unexpectedly loses their job. At first, the shock can feel overwhelming. The immediate uncertainty brings not only financial stress but also self-doubt, prompting one to question their abilities and worth. For many, the first few weeks may be filled with complex feelings—fear, anxiety, and frustration. It may seem like the end of the road, and the future appears clouded and unclear.

However, for some, this difficult experience sparks the beginning of a new chapter. Instead of seeing the job loss as an irreversible setback, they start to look inward and ask, *What do I truly want from my career? What passions have I neglected or ignored?* Through self-reflection, support from others, and tapping into their inner resilience, they begin to see the situation not as a roadblock but as an opportunity to explore new possibilities. Some may go back to school, acquire new skills, or pursue a passion they had put on hold for years. Others might start their own businesses or shift to careers that align more closely with their personal values and interests.

Though the path may not be easy, many find that this difficult moment leads them to a life that feels more fulfilling and authentic, reigniting a sense of purpose that they had long forgotten. The journey of rediscovery becomes a powerful testament to resilience—the ability to embrace change, learn from adversity, and find new meaning in the face of life's challenges.

Other instances include overcoming personal traumas such as divorce or the death of a loved one. In these scenarios, resilience manifests as the capacity to grieve appropriately while actively seeking support systems that may include friends, family, and mental health professionals. The process of grieving is not linear; it can involve a whirlwind of emotions, from deep sadness to moments of anger and confusion. Resilient individuals allow themselves to feel these emotions without judgment, recognizing that each stage is an important part of the healing journey.

As they progress through this difficult terrain, resilience enables individuals to reflect on their experiences, leading to meaningful personal insights. Over time, they begin to integrate these experiences into their lives, converting the raw pain into moments of introspection and emotional growth. Resilience, thus, becomes a fundamental tool in life, allowing individuals to endure their traumas and emerge stronger and more empathetic toward others facing similar challenges.

However, building resilience is often hindered by common obstacles, such as the fear of failure. This fear can act as a significant barrier, preventing individuals from taking necessary risks and stepping out of their comfort zones. Recognizing and confronting this fear can create pathways toward resilience. Acknowledging that failure is a natural part of life and a potential catalyst for growth helps individuals become more comfortable with setbacks as temporary stages on the path to achieving their goals.

Guidance on overcoming these barriers can be invaluable. For instance, developing a growth mindset—a belief that abilities can improve over time—can significantly enhance resilience (Hurley, 2024). Viewing failures as opportunities for growth rather than signs of inadequacy creates an environment where individuals feel safe to experiment and innovate, which encourages both personal and emotional development.

Principles like gratitude, compassion, acceptance, meaning, and forgiveness help individuals interpret life events in a more positive light and support emotional healing. Nurturing these attributes is important for building resilience. These principles shape thoughts and actions, creating a strong foundation from which to view challenges not as insurmountable obstacles but as vital steps in personal growth.

Resilience isn't solely a personal endeavor. Social connections play an important role in resilience-building efforts. Close ties with family, friends, and communities offer a sense of belonging and security. They provide the scaffolding needed during tough times, enabling individuals to lean on others for support, wisdom, and different perspectives.

DEVELOPING A GROWTH MINDSET

A growth mindset represents a powerful approach that empowers you by promoting resilience and enabling you to confront life's challenges with confidence. When you begin to see obstacles as opportunities for growth instead of insurmountable barriers, you can completely alter the way you handle challenges and setbacks. Those who embody a growth mindset are motivated to learn and enhance themselves through hardship, resisting the temptation to succumb to failure, which ultimately ensures greater resilience.

Imagine facing a life-altering situation, like being diagnosed with a serious illness or experiencing a major personal loss. In the face of overwhelming uncertainty, maintaining a growth mindset might sound like telling yourself, *This is incredibly hard, but I can use this experience to grow stronger and learn more about myself.* This shift in perspective allows you to see that, although the road ahead is full of challenges, each moment presents an opportunity to build resilience and develop new ways of coping. Instead of letting despair take over, you're motivated to explore different approaches to healing or overcoming the obstacle, gradually increasing your ability to face future difficulties with courage and a deeper understanding of your own strength.

A vital technique within this mindset is reframing negative thoughts. Negative self-talk often limits our progress and resilience, but by consciously shifting these thoughts into opportunities for growth, we can strengthen our emotional resilience. For example, instead of saying, "I failed; I'm not good enough," you might reframe it to, "I've learned what doesn't work, and now I can try a new approach." Reframing shows that mistakes aren't final but rather stepping stones to success, encouraging resilience and motivating perseverance.

Feedback plays a pivotal role in strengthening a growth mindset. It serves as a mirror reflecting areas where improvement is possible and provides invaluable insights into personal development. Embracing feedback allows for continuous growth. Constructive criticism should be viewed not as a hit to your self-esteem but as valuable guidance for improvement. For example, if a teacher suggests refining an essay, seize this as an opportunity to enhance your writing skills. Regularly reflecting on such feedback helps you recognize growth and adjust your approach, reinforcing resilience over time.

Celebrating small achievements is another cornerstone of developing a growth mindset. Acknowledging progress, no matter how minor, fuels motivation and builds confidence. Consider the effort required to master a musical instrument or learn a new language. Recognizing and celebrating incremental successes along the journey, such as mastering a chord on the guitar or having a basic conversation in French, keeps you motivated to continue your efforts. This habit affirms your progress and reinforces the understanding that growth is a process, helping to build resilience when faced with larger challenges.

Despite the practical benefits of adopting a growth mindset, it's important to remember that cultural and societal pressures can sometimes glorify innate talent over effort, potentially discouraging persistence. Breaking free from these societal norms is important. Surrounding yourself with like-minded individuals who value effort and learning can inspire you to persist. Additionally, celebrating stories of those who attribute their success to hard work and resilience rather than natural talent can reinforce your commitment to maintaining a growth mindset.

However, achieving a sustained growth mindset requires intentional effort. Here are some guidelines to help nurture this mindset effectively:

- **Recognize the power of beliefs:** Our beliefs shape how we approach challenges and setbacks. Understand that abilities are not fixed but can evolve with time, effort, and perseverance. Take time to reflect on your current beliefs and actively work to replace those that limit your potential with more empowering, growth-oriented thoughts. A shift in mindset starts with the recognition that growth is within reach for anyone willing to put in the work.

- **Embrace challenges:** Growth occurs outside of our comfort zones. Actively seek out situations that challenge your abilities and push you to grow. When faced with obstacles, resilience helps build adaptability and inner strength. Instead of avoiding difficulties, see them as opportunities to expand your skills and expand your boundaries.

- **Learn from criticism:** Constructive criticism is not an attack on your abilities but a tool for improvement. View feedback as an essential part of your learning process. Regularly ask for input from others, whether it's from colleagues, mentors, or peers, and use it to refine your skills and strategies. Approaching feedback with an open mind allows you to identify areas of improvement and take actionable steps toward growth.

- **Celebrate effort, not just outcomes:** Shift your focus from solely celebrating final results to appreciating the effort put into the process. Acknowledge that growth happens through persistence, hard work, and dedication, not just through achieving goals. Break large objectives into smaller, manageable milestones and take the time to celebrate each step forward. Recognizing effort reinforces the belief that progress is the result of consistent, intentional action.

- **Seek diverse perspectives:** Challenging your own thinking is vital for personal growth. Expose yourself to ideas and viewpoints that differ from your own to expand your perspective. Being open to new insights and learning from others helps break down cognitive biases and promotes flexibility. This openness to diverse perspectives nurtures a richer, more adaptive mindset that can easily adjust to changing situations.

- **Practice self-care:** A sustainable growth mindset requires both mental and physical well-being. Prioritize activities that nourish your body and mind, such as regular exercise, sufficient rest, and mindfulness practices. When you prioritize your overall health, you maintain the energy and focus necessary to stay motivated and engaged in the growth process. Self-care is not a luxury; it's an integral part of staying resilient and committed to long-term growth.

EMOTIONAL REGULATION TECHNIQUES

Managing emotions can often feel like trying to steer a ship through turbulent waters. For individuals of all ages, it's essential to have effective methods for handling overwhelming emotions constructively. Identifying these emotions is the first vital step in gaining control over them. Just like naming an unfamiliar sea allows sailors to map their journey, recognizing and naming your feelings helps you respond to them more healthily.

Reflect on times when you've felt overwhelmed. What was happening in those moments? Were there specific triggers, such as certain people or situations, that intensified your emotions? Keeping a mood journal can be a valuable tool in this process. It helps track moments when emotions run high and allows you to identify recurring patterns. Recognizing your unique emotional triggers equips you with the ability to approach life's challenges with greater calm and clarity. Identifying and managing these triggers strengthens resilience, improving your capacity to respond thoughtfully to stressors and tackle challenges with increased ease and flexibility (*10 Effective Strategies*, n.d.).

MOOD JOURNALING EXERCISES

Evaluate your mood by shading the block, with one indicating a very poor day and five representing an excellent day.

1	2	3	4	5

Here are three mood journaling prompts to help evaluate how you feel about your day:

How am I feeling right now, and what do I think is contributing to this mood? Here are some options for how you may be feeling:

- **Happy:** a positive, joyful state; feeling upbeat and excited
- **Motivated:** feeling driven and clear-headed, with a strong sense of determination
- **Anxious:** a feeling of stress or unease due to pressure or uncertainty
- **Frustrated:** a sense of annoyance or impatience caused by obstacles or setbacks
- **Calm:** a peaceful, relaxed state; feeling at ease in the present moment
- **Sad or lonely**: emotional distress or isolation, often due to loss or disconnection
- **Drained:** a lack of energy or inspiration, leading to exhaustion or apathy
- **Guilty:** emotional discomfort or remorse related to past actions or decisions

_____

_____

_____

_____

_____

_____

_____

_____

_____

_____

_____

_____

_____

_____

What is something I can do to improve or shift my mood today?

_____

_____

_____

_____

_____

_____

_____

_____

_____

_____

_____

_____

_____

_____

What moments stood out as either positive or negative?

_____

_____

_____

_____

_____

_____

_____

_____

_____

_____

_____

_____

_____

Once you've identified your emotions, having strategies at your disposal can significantly help. Journaling is one such technique that offers immediate relief by providing an outlet for your feelings. Writing down thoughts and emotions can serve as a release, helping clear your mind. Additionally, physical activities like jogging or cycling can channel your energy in a positive direction, while deep breathing exercises can help calm your nervous system, encouraging relaxation during emotional turmoil. Picture a storm calming as the waves gradually settle; these techniques act as anchors, steadying your emotional state.

Puzzles and Emotions

Engaging with puzzles serves as an effective method for emotional regulation. Solving puzzles fosters concentration and mindfulness, redirecting focus from stress to a soothing, goal-directed activity. Additionally, puzzles demand critical thinking and problem-solving abilities, instilling a sense of accomplishment that enhances self-esteem. As individuals explore the task, they often achieve a reflective state of mind, enabling clearer processing of emotions and thoughts. The physical interaction with tangible puzzles also heightens sensory involvement, anchoring individuals in the present and fostering tranquility. This method improves your ability to concentrate, cope with stress, and face challenges with a serene and clear mindset, enhancing your emotional resilience and helping you to adjust to tough situations.

Support Networks

Building a support network is equally important. Just as a sturdy net catches a falling trapeze artist, having trusted friends and mentors provides safety during emotional free falls. Engaging with friends or mentors who understand and support your emotional journey can offer perspective and comfort in times of need. They act as sounding boards, allowing you to express your feelings openly. Communication is essential in maintaining these relationships. Regularly checking in with your support network strengthens bonds and ensures you have allies ready to catch you when life feels overwhelming.

Preparing for Triggers

Planning ahead for potential emotional triggers can give you a valuable edge. Anticipating stressful situations allows you to rehearse coping strategies before they occur. Techniques like the "Cope Ahead" strategy from dialectical behavior therapy (DBT) help prepare your mind, promoting composure when intense emotions arise (CounselorAid, 2024). Visualizing your response and practicing how to handle certain scenarios is similar to rehearsing lines for a play. Having a clear plan boosts confidence and reduces anxiety when facing emotionally charged situations. Implementing this proactive approach fosters resilience, reduces stress, and boosts your ability to handle emotionally charged situations.

Setting Boundaries

The power of boundaries shouldn't be underestimated either. Setting limits with people or circumstances that consistently trigger negative emotions is sometimes necessary to protect your mental well-being. Imagine boundaries as the protective walls of a castle—they guard you against unnecessary distress. It's okay to minimize contact with individuals who drain your emotional reserves or avoid topics that spark anxiety. These boundaries aren't about cutting off connections but rather about creating healthy spaces where you can thrive emotionally. Setting boundaries builds resilience by protecting your mental well-being from negative triggers, allowing you to create healthy spaces for emotional growth and strength. This will be further discussed in Chapter 6.

Positive Coping Skills

Integrating positive coping skills into your daily routine significantly enhances emotional management. Whether it's engaging in art, music, or sports, these activities redirect your focus and provide emotional resilience. Think of these coping skills as tools in your toolkit, ready to be used whenever you need them. They allow you to transform stress into creative expression, turning potentially destructive energy into something constructive and rewarding.

Professional Help

Finally, never hesitate to seek professional support if needed. Sometimes talking with a counselor or therapist can illuminate new paths through complex emotions. Professionals provide guidance tailored to your individual needs, offering strategies that might not occur to you otherwise. They help reinforce the skills you're developing, ensuring you're never truly alone in your emotional journey (*10 Effective Strategies*, n.d.).

OVERCOMING SETBACKS AND ADVERSITY

Developing emotional resilience is an essential capability that every adult should acquire to effectively navigate life's challenges and transitions. One impactful approach to strengthening resilience is transforming obstacles into opportunities for personal growth and understanding. Instead of viewing obstacles as insurmountable barriers, see them as stepping stones to greater knowledge and personal growth. Embracing this mindset encourages a proactive approach, allowing individuals to persevere despite difficulties. Take, for example, a professional who faces challenges in a significant project. Rather than succumbing to despair, they could use the setback to identify weak areas, refine their strategies, and ultimately improve future performance.

A vital component of emotional resilience is the use of effective coping strategies in times of stress. One powerful technique is positive self-talk, which helps reinforce confidence by highlighting strengths and cultivating empowering beliefs about oneself. For example, reminding yourself of previous successes or affirming your abilities before a challenging task, such as delivering a speech, can help reduce anxiety and improve performance. Additionally, strong problem-solving skills are essential for building resilience. When confronted with a challenge, breaking it down into smaller, more manageable tasks allows individuals to tackle each part methodically, promoting a sense of control and boosting confidence in their ability to navigate difficult situations (Hurley, 2024).

A supportive community is also important when facing tough times. Reaching out for help during difficult moments helps manage stress and strengthens relationships through shared experiences. Whether it's turning to family, friends, or mentors, having someone to confide in can provide fresh perspectives and emotional comfort. For example, a teenager coping with the loss of a loved one may find that talking with trusted individuals lightens their emotional load and encourages healing. Additionally, connecting with support groups or networks allows people to bond over similar challenges, creating a sense of belonging and reducing feelings of isolation.

Adapting to changes and remaining flexible are key components of building a resilient mindset. Life is unpredictable, and the ability to adjust to new realities ensures smoother transitions through various life stages. This adaptability involves openness to different possibilities and a willingness to alter plans when necessary. For example, if a planned career path becomes infeasible, exploring alternative avenues rather than fixating on the original plan demonstrates flexibility. This flexibility enables individuals to face life's uncertainties with assurance, transforming unforeseen changes into opportunities for personal development (*Overcoming Obstacles*, n.d.).

Guidelines can be incredibly helpful in handling life's challenges, as specific coping strategies provide clear pathways to build resilience. Engaging in activities like knitting allows you to reflect on your feelings and experiences, helping you identify patterns and understand your emotions more effectively, leading to healthier responses. Regular physical activity, whether it's a simple walk or a more intense workout, reduces stress and boosts mood, complementing the calming effects of knitting. Additionally, seeking support during adversity plays a crucial role in resilience. Establishing a reliable support network grants access to advice, encouragement, and diverse perspectives when facing difficulties. Reaching out to others prevents feelings of isolation, often associated with challenging situations, cultivating a sense of community and shared resilience. Conversations with trustworthy individuals can reveal insights or solutions that may have been previously overlooked, emphasizing the power of connection during trying times.

How Parents and Educators Can Help

Educators and parents play a pivotal role in empowering children and students to develop emotional resilience by modeling the behaviors and mindsets that encourage growth in the face of adversity. One key approach is to encourage a mindset that views obstacles as opportunities for growth rather than insurmountable barriers. By demonstrating how to overcome challenges, whether through adjusting strategies or learning from mistakes, adults can teach children to embrace difficulties as part of the learning process. For example, parents can guide children through frustrations in schoolwork by helping them break down tasks into smaller, more manageable steps, reinforcing the idea that setbacks are temporary and can be used to improve future performance.

Additionally, positive self-talk and problem-solving skills can be nurtured through consistent encouragement and reinforcement. Educators can create a supportive classroom environment where students are reminded of their past successes, helping to build confidence and a sense of competence. When children struggle with assignments or social challenges, parents can reinforce empowering language, such as "You can handle this" or "Let's figure out a new approach together."

Finally, creating a strong support system is essential for cultivating emotional resilience. Parents and educators can encourage students to seek help when needed and establish networks of support, both in and outside the classroom. Whether through peer groups, mentoring, or family discussions, having someone to confide in during tough times helps reduce feelings of isolation and promotes emotional growth. By modeling these behaviors and providing the tools necessary for self-regulation and support, educators and parents empower children to build resilience, adapt to life's changes, and thrive in the face of challenges.

As we move into Chapter 4, "Fostering Self-Awareness," we will examine how self-awareness is necessary for developing resilience. It shifts the focus from managing challenges to understanding how recognizing our thoughts and emotions aids personal growth and self-acceptance. The chapter shares techniques like mind mapping, values clarification, and feedback to align actions with values and manage emotions effectively. Identifying emotional responses during stressful situations enhances resilience, while comprehending personal values nurtures authenticity.

KEY TAKEAWAYS

- Developing emotional resilience is essential for handling challenges at different stages of life, allowing individuals to recover from setbacks while maintaining their mental well-being.

- Resilience is the ability to adapt to adversity and stress, leading to personal growth and emotional stability.

- The benefits of resilience include better emotional regulation, improved coping skills, and the ability to see challenges as opportunities for learning and growth.

- Building resilience often involves adopting a growth mindset, which encourages viewing failures as opportunities for improvement and personal development.

- Effective emotional regulation techniques include identifying and managing emotional triggers, practicing positive self-talk, and using healthy coping strategies such as journaling and physical activities.

- A supportive community is vital for resilience, as social connections provide emotional comfort, new perspectives, and a sense of belonging during tough times.

- As individuals build resilience, they learn to embrace change and flexibility, turning obstacles into opportunities for personal growth and understanding.

CHAPTER 4

Fostering Self-Awareness

Identifying our personal triggers gives us the power to control our emotional reactions, enabling us to face life's challenges with courage, clarity, and purpose.

B uilding self-awareness is a vital step in understanding who we are and what drives us. It is essential for personal growth and self-acceptance, as it enables us to recognize our thoughts, emotions, and reactions. When we tune in to ourselves, we start a journey of self-discovery, uncovering the layers that make up who we are. This is important for individuals going through emotional challenges, as it provides tools to better handle life's ups and downs. Support from family and friends can help strengthen emotional resilience by encouraging self-awareness. For educators and wellness practitioners, nurturing this skill across all age groups helps develop emotional intelligence, empowering individuals to face challenges with confidence.

SELF-REFLECTION TECHNIQUES

Understanding Oneself for Personal Development

Understanding oneself is essential for personal development and self-acceptance. One effective method to initiate this process of introspection is through mind mapping. Establishing a consistent time for mind mapping helps make it a regular habit. Choose a comfortable setting where you can focus without distractions. Start with a central idea or question, such as your core values or recent impactful experiences, and let your thoughts branch out naturally. Use colors, symbols, or images to enhance clarity and creativity. These strategies help organize your thoughts visually, uncover patterns, and build a deeper understanding of yourself, aiding in personal growth and acceptance.

Values Clarification

Values clarification is a powerful tool for encouraging self-awareness and aligning actions with personal principles. This practice encourages intentional reflection on core values, creating space to evaluate how these values influence decisions and behaviors. By identifying and prioritizing what truly matters, individuals gain clarity and develop a stronger sense of purpose. Begin by sitting comfortably in a quiet space, focusing on a specific value or question, such as "What drives my decisions?" or "What principles guide my relationships?" Let your thoughts emerge naturally, exploring their connections to your daily life. Over time, clarifying your values becomes a meaningful practice for deepening self-understanding, aligning actions with beliefs, and managing challenges with authenticity and confidence. Regular reflection offers a pathway to living a life that resonates with your deepest convictions.

Gaining Insights From Others

Gaining insights from others is essential for enhancing self-awareness. Often, we have blind spots that hinder our personal growth. Feedback from trusted friends, family members, or mentors can illuminate these areas. Constructive criticism can highlight areas for improvement, offering a clearer picture of how others perceive us, which may differ from our self-perception. Receive feedback with an open mind and curiosity rather than defensiveness. Ask targeted questions to gather specific insights and use this external perspective to uncover areas for personal growth. Embracing feedback encourages a mindset of ongoing learning and self-improvement, offering valuable insights into yourself that might otherwise go unnoticed. The goal is not just to hear the feedback but to reflect on it and incorporate the insights into your self-awareness.

Prompted Reflection Through Targeted Questions

Prompted reflection through targeted questions is another method to stimulate introspection. Asking yourself questions like "What are my core values?" encourages deep self-assessment. When you explore such questions thoughtfully, you might uncover those principles most integral to your identity. Recognizing these values allows you to align your actions and decisions accordingly, promoting authenticity in your life. Take time to contemplate each question genuinely, allowing revelations to emerge naturally. These questions act as catalysts for powerful realizations about who you are and what matters most to you. Having a clear awareness of your values and beliefs guides your choices and empowers you to live more authentically, aligning your life with your true essence.

Tools for Young Individuals

For young individuals grappling with emotional challenges, like teens and young adults, these introspective tools are invaluable. They offer methods for channeling emotions constructively, thereby building a framework for better understanding oneself. Additionally, parents and guardians can use these techniques to support their children's emotional growth, encouraging open dialogue about feelings and thoughts. Educators and wellness practitioners might find these strategies beneficial for guiding youth and encouraging emotional intelligence and resilience within educational settings.

SELF-REFLECTION EXERCISE: CORE VALUES EXPLORATION

Purpose

This exercise aims to guide you in identifying and reflecting on your core values, helping you align your actions and decisions with what truly matters to you and fostering authenticity in your life.

INSTRUCTIONS

Take some time to thoughtfully answer the following questions. Reflect on your answers and let them guide your understanding of your personal values.

What qualities do I admire most in others?

The traits you admire in others often reflect the values you hold dear. Whether it's kindness, ambition, honesty, or creativity, these qualities can reveal what you truly value in relationships and interactions.

_____

_____

_____

_____

_____

_____

_____

_____

_____

_____

_____

_____

_____

_____

_____

_____

_____

- **Suggestion:** If you're unsure about the qualities you admire in others, think about your friends, family, or celebrities you look up to. What do they do that makes them stand out to you? Do they help others, work hard, or stand up for what's right? It's okay if you're not sure right away; these qualities can show up in small ways that matter to you.
- **Example:** Maybe you admire someone for being super kind, or you appreciate a friend's determination to stick with something even when it's tough. These are signs of qualities like kindness, perseverance, and empathy, which could be your core values.

When have I felt the most proud of myself?

What values were reflected in that moment?

Pride often comes from living in alignment with your core values. Reflecting on the moments that made you feel proud can help you pinpoint the values that drive your sense of accomplishment.

_____

_____

_____

_____

_____

_____

_____

_____

_____

_____

_____

_____

_____

_____

_____

_____

_____

_____

_____

_____

_____

- **Suggestion:** Think about times when you've accomplished something, no matter how small, and felt really good about it. Maybe you helped a friend, finished a big project, or stood up for what's right. These proud moments often show what values matter most to you.
- **Example:** If you've ever felt proud of helping a teammate or standing up for a friend, that could reflect values like loyalty, teamwork, and kindness. These moments can give you a clue about what's important to you.

What would I never compromise on, regardless of the situation?

The things you're unwilling to budge on are the most nonnegotiable parts of your identity. Whether it's honesty, loyalty, or fairness, this question helps you identify values you hold sacred.

_____

_____

_____

_____

_____

_____

_____

_____

_____

_____

- **Suggestion:** If you're unsure what you'd never compromise on, think about times when you've faced peer pressure or tough decisions. Did you ever stand up for something even though it wasn't an easy choice? These situations can show you what values you hold most strongly.
- **Example:** Maybe you would never compromise on being honest with your friends, or you refuse to go along with something you think is wrong. This reflects values like honesty, integrity, and fairness.

If I could focus on one priority in my life, what would that be and why?
This question forces you to distill what matters most to you. It challenges you to think about the one thing that drives your decisions, whether it's family, personal growth, or making a positive impact.

_____

_____

_____

_____

_____

_____

_____

_____

_____

_____

_____

_____

_____

_____

_____

_____

_____

_____

_____

_____

_____

_____

_____

- **Suggestion:** If you're not sure what you'd prioritize, think about what makes you happy or what you want to achieve in the future. Whether it's your friendships, school success, or something you love doing, the things you care about most can show you what matters to you.
- **Example:** If you're really passionate about helping others, you might prioritize making a positive impact. Or, if you value personal growth, maybe learning and improving yourself is your top priority.

What do I find myself consistently standing up for?

When you find yourself advocating for something, it's often because it aligns with your core values. This could include standing up for equality, personal freedom, or environmental sustainability.

_____

_____

_____

_____

_____

_____

_____

_____

_____

_____

- **Suggestion:** Think about times when you've spoken up or defended someone or something. Do you stand up for your friends, fairness, or the environment? These situations often show what values matter most to you and what you're willing to fight for.
- **Example:** If you find yourself standing up for a classmate who's being treated unfairly, that shows you value fairness and empathy. If you're passionate about the environment, you might be an advocate for sustainability.

When do I feel most authentic to myself?

Authenticity comes from living in accordance with your values. Reflecting on when you feel most yourself can help you understand the environment, actions, and decisions that allow your true self to shine.

_____

_____

_____

_____

_____

_____

_____

_____

_____

_____

_____

_____

_____

_____

_____

_____

_____

_____

_____

_____

_____

_____

_____

- **Suggestion:** If you're not sure when you feel most like yourself, think about times when you felt at ease and comfortable. Were you with close friends, doing something you love, or standing up for what's right? These moments usually reflect when you're aligned with your values.
- **Example:** If you feel most authentic when you're helping others or participating in activities you enjoy, that could mean those things are aligned with your values, like kindness, teamwork, or creativity.

What role does integrity play in my decisions?

Integrity is a fundamental aspect of many people's core values. This question helps you evaluate the importance you place on honesty and transparency in your decisions and how these values shape your actions and behavior.

_____

_____

_____

_____

_____

_____

_____

_____

_____

_____

_____

_____

_____

_____

_____

_____

_____

_____

_____

_____

_____

_____

- **Suggestion:** If you're unsure how integrity impacts your decisions, think about moments when you had to choose between doing what's right or doing what's easy. Making the right choice might not always be easy, but it shows you value honesty, trust, and doing the right thing, even when it's hard.
- **Example:** If you've ever decided not to cheat on a test, even though you knew it could be easier, that reflects integrity. It shows that you value honesty, even in tough situations.

How do I want others to describe me?

What values do I want them to associate with me?

This question asks you to think about the impression you leave on others. The traits you wish to be known for—such as being reliable, compassionate, or innovative—are often tied to your core values.

_____

_____

_____

_____

_____

_____

_____

_____

_____

_____

_____

_____

_____

_____

_____

_____

_____

_____

_____

_____

_____

- **Suggestion:** If you're unsure how you want others to describe you, think about qualities you admire in people. What traits do you hope others see in you? Whether it's kindness, reliability, or creativity, this can help guide you in identifying the values you want to be known for.
- **Example:** Maybe you hope others describe you as trustworthy and caring. If so, that might reflect values like reliability, loyalty, and kindness.

RECOGNIZING PERSONAL TRIGGERS

Recognizing personal triggers that influence emotional responses and behavior is an important step in developing self-awareness. Understanding how external stimuli connect to our internal reactions helps improve emotional management, allowing for more thoughtful and balanced responses. A useful approach to identifying these triggers is through self-observation of emotional reactions. This practice encourages individuals to notice when their emotions are intensified and reflect on the situations that may have contributed to those feelings.

The Impact of Political Discussions

For example, imagine having a conversation with a close friend, and during the discussion, you suddenly feel a surge of anger when they express political views that strongly differ from your own. By taking a moment to pause and reflect on this emotional reaction, you may recognize that these political discussions tend to trigger your anger because of deeply held beliefs or past experiences tied to those views. Understanding this pattern enables you to anticipate similar reactions in future conversations and prepares you to respond more thoughtfully. Instead of reacting impulsively, you could choose to calmly express your perspective, set boundaries around political discussions if needed, or redirect the conversation toward common ground. This self-observation process helps you manage emotional responses responsibly and encourages personal growth by fostering awareness of the triggers behind your anger (wadmin, 2024a).

The Influence of the Environment

Furthermore, becoming aware of how different environments or interactions affect your energy levels can provide valuable insights into your personal alignments and necessary changes. Each individual resonates differently with various settings, people, and activities. For instance, being in crowded spaces may drain some individuals, while others thrive in social scenarios. Reflecting on these experiences helps pinpoint which environments energize or deplete you, allowing you to make adjustments for your well-being.

Imagine feeling especially tired after spending time in a busy café. Recognizing that this happens to you can encourage you to choose quieter environments, helping you stay mentally and emotionally balanced. On the other hand, if you feel energized after group activities, you can prioritize these experiences to keep your energy levels up. This awareness empowers you to make better decisions, shaping a lifestyle that aligns with your needs and goals, ultimately boosting your emotional resilience (wadmin, 2024b).

Evaluating Behavior Under Stress

Evaluating behavior patterns during periods of stress also reveals areas for growth and aids in managing expectations and developing coping strategies. Stress often magnifies existing behavioral tendencies, making it an opportune moment to observe and understand how we react under pressure. Examining these patterns helps us pinpoint recurring issues that impede personal growth, allowing us to find suitable solutions.

Consider how stress might impact your work performance or relationships. During tight deadlines, you may notice a tendency to withdraw from colleagues or become overly critical of your own efforts. Acknowledging these behaviors allows you to develop targeted strategies for improvement, such as practicing open communication or setting realistic goals. This helps set healthier expectations for yourself and others, minimizing stress-related conflicts and supporting overall well-being.

Recognizing Physical Symptoms

Recognizing physical symptoms like tension or fatigue serves as an important alert to reassess emotional states and improve overall well-being. Physical manifestations of emotional stress, such as headaches or muscle tension, often signal unresolved emotional triggers (wadmin, 2024b). Developing an awareness of these symptoms enhances self-awareness and empowers individuals to take proactive measures for their mental health.

For example, you might experience tension across your shoulders whenever you encounter a particularly stressful situation at work. Recognizing this physical sign allows you to explore its emotional origins and pinpoint the aspects of your work environment that trigger such a response. With this awareness, you can explore relaxation techniques or seek professional guidance to address the underlying causes, ultimately improving both physical and emotional health (wadmin, 2024b).

Utilizing Self-Observation

To effectively utilize self-observation as a tool, consider maintaining a diary to track emotional reactions and corresponding triggers. Write down instances when your emotions feel heightened, along with details about the context and any specific stimuli involved. Over time, reviewing these entries can unveil patterns and provide clarity about your emotional landscape.

This practice encourages a deeper understanding of your personal triggers and paves the way for more intentional emotional management. Recording these observations creates a valuable resource for reflection, providing insights into recurring patterns and enabling you to make intentional decisions about how to respond to different situations This type of introspection promotes personal growth and greater self-acceptance, leading to a more balanced and harmonious relationship with your emotions.

Overall, creating self-awareness through the identification of emotional triggers is essential for personal growth and well-being. By engaging in self-observation and reflecting on emotional reactions, individuals gain valuable insights into their triggers, enabling them to manage emotions more responsibly. Understanding how different environments and interactions influence energy levels further informs decisions that align with personal needs.

UNDERSTANDING PERSONAL VALUES

Understanding and identifying one's core values is an important step in ensuring self-awareness and personal growth. Core values are the guiding principles that shape our behavior, decisions, and self-understanding. Exploring these values allows individuals to develop authenticity, integrity, and resilience.

Identifying your core values can lead to significant personal growth, and one effective method for achieving this is through a personal SWOT analysis—evaluating your Strengths, Weaknesses, Opportunities, and Threats. Begin by exploring your strengths, such as traits that reflect your values, like compassion, honesty, or resilience, and how these qualities positively influence your decisions. Next, examine your weaknesses—areas where your behavior or choices may fall short of the values you aspire to uphold, such as struggles with consistency or setting boundaries. Opportunities come into focus as you identify ways to live more authentically, whether by nurturing meaningful relationships, pursuing fulfilling goals, or contributing to causes aligned with your beliefs. Finally, assess threats, such as external pressures, self-doubt, or habits that may pull you away from your values. By taking this comprehensive approach, you gain a clearer understanding of what matters most, enabling you to make intentional, values-driven decisions that shape a purposeful and aligned life.

Reflecting on how well your actions align with your identified values is another fundamental aspect of ensuring self-awareness. This reflection encourages individuals to live authentically, where their actions resonate with their inner beliefs. It can also highlight discrepancies, which often cause stress or discomfort when there's a misalignment. For example, if someone values family but consistently prioritizes work over spending time with loved ones, this misalignment can lead to feelings of guilt or dissatisfaction. Regularly evaluating whether our actions support our core values helps maintain integrity and reduces internal conflict (Perry, 2023).

Recognizing that our values can evolve over time is essential for navigating life's transitions with adaptability and clarity. As people grow and experience different life stages, what was once important may change, giving rise to new values that better fit current realities. For example, a young adult's priority might shift from professional achievement to health and well-being as they mature. Understanding that value evolution is natural allows for greater flexibility and reduces confusion when faced with changes. It serves as a reminder that self-awareness is a continuous journey, requiring regular introspection to remain true to oneself.

Engaging with the community or its cultural values can further deepen one's understanding of personal beliefs and identity. Observing and interacting with the values prevalent within one's cultural background or community can provide insights into external influences shaping personal values. Whether it's the importance of community service or the value of family traditions, these societal norms have a significant influence on individual beliefs. Acknowledging and reflecting on how collective values influence personal ones helps individuals gain a broader perspective on their identity and the diverse influences shaping their experiences.

Creating a safe space for open discussions with peers or mentors about personal values can help facilitate these explorations. Sharing perspectives often uncovers new insights or reinforces existing beliefs. Engaging in community activities also provides practical experiences that deepen your understanding of both personal and communal values.

SETTING REALISTIC PERSONAL GOALS

Self-awareness is a powerful tool for personal growth. It involves understanding your emotions, motivations, and values, helping you make choices that align with your authentic self. When you cultivate self-awareness, you gain clarity about what truly matters, empowering you to set goals that resonate with your priorities. This not only enhances decision-making but also strengthens your ability to stay committed to your objectives.

Setting goals that align with your personal values and self-awareness can lead to significant transformation in your life. One of the most effective ways to do this is by using the SMART criteria, a widely recognized framework for goal setting. SMART stands for Specific, Measurable, Achievable, Relevant, and Time-Bound, and it provides a clear, structured approach to setting goals. These elements help ensure your goals are focused and actionable, making it easier to track progress. For example, instead of a vague goal like "be healthier," a SMART goal would specify, "exercise for 30 minutes, five days a week, over the next month." This provides a clear direction and measurable steps, which can help maintain motivation and drive (*SMART Goals*, n.d.).

Setting goals involves anticipating potential challenges. Obstacles are inevitable, but identifying them early helps you prepare to face them without frustration. Recognizing possible setbacks, such as time constraints, lack of resources, or self-doubt, enables you to develop effective strategies for overcoming them. This approach strengthens your problem-solving skills, allowing you to adjust your tactics rather than abandoning your goals when difficulties arise.

A potent ally in pursuing your objectives is the role of accountability partners. Involving someone else in your journey toward achieving your goals adds layers of motivation and commitment, providing a supportive network that encourages collaborative growth. This could be a friend, mentor, or support group that shares or understands your ambitions. When you know someone else is invested in your success, it becomes a shared pursuit, creating a sense of responsibility and inspiration to follow through.

Cultivating self-awareness is an enlightening journey that establishes the foundation for personal development, emotional strength, and self-acceptance. The techniques outlined in this chapter enable individuals to achieve a deep understanding of their thoughts, emotions, and actions. These practices encourage authenticity, improve emotional regulation, and empower individuals to align their behaviors with their fundamental values. Approaching self-awareness as a continuous journey nurtures a more harmonious relationship with ourselves and others, resulting in a balanced and fulfilling life.

While self-awareness is the foundation of personal growth, self-acceptance brings it to life by helping us embrace every aspect of who we are. In a world often influenced by societal pressures and external expectations, developing self-acceptance requires intentionality and compassion. In the next chapter, we will explore practical strategies for overcoming societal pressures, promoting body positivity, celebrating individuality, and practicing self-compassion. This chapter will invite you to challenge limiting narratives, honor your unique journey, and build a foundation of inner peace and self-love that supports lasting personal fulfillment.

KEY TAKEAWAYS

- Developing self-awareness is crucial for personal growth and self-acceptance, helping individuals recognize their thoughts, emotions, and reactions.

- Self-reflection techniques like mind mapping and values clarification guide individuals in discovering their core values, leading to more intentional decision-making.

- Feedback from trusted friends and mentors can shed light on blind spots, deepen self-awareness, and support continuous learning and self-improvement.

- Reflective questions prompt introspection, helping individuals understand their identity and align their actions with their core values.

- Identifying personal triggers and behavioral patterns helps individuals manage emotions effectively and respond more thoughtfully to stressors.

- Performing a personal SWOT analysis allows individuals to examine their strengths, weaknesses, opportunities, and threats, offering clarity for making values-driven decisions.

- Setting realistic personal goals using the SMART criteria ensures that goals are specific, measurable, achievable, relevant, and time-bound, boosting motivation and commitment.

- Engaging in open conversations about personal values and experiences, while maintaining accountability partnerships, promotes deeper understanding and encourages growth.

CHAPTER 5

Cultivating Self-Acceptance

Our value isn't determined by societal expectations,
but by the love and acceptance we show ourselves.

Embracing self-acceptance is an essential journey that requires us to examine how our sense of self relates to external societal expectations. In today's world, external expectations often dictate rigid definitions of beauty, success, and worth, creating an environment where individuals feel compelled to conform to narrow standards in order to fit in. These prescribed ideals can erode self-confidence and cloud the ability to fully appreciate one's unique qualities. As you read through this chapter, take time to reflect on how these societal expectations have influenced your perception of yourself and others. Recognizing their impact is the first step toward breaking free from the limitations of these unrealistic ideals.

OVERCOMING SOCIETAL PRESSURES

In our pursuit of self-acceptance, it's important to take a closer look at societal standards and how they impact us. Society often sets benchmarks that are not only challenging but sometimes unattainable, creating unrealistic expectations. Whether it's the image of perfect beauty portrayed in the media or the idea of success defined by material wealth and status, these standards can lead individuals, especially teens and young adults, to feel inadequate when they aren't met. This feeling of inadequacy can become deeply ingrained, eroding a person's self-esteem and mental well-being (Michot, 2023).

Recognizing the societal pressures we encounter is an essential first step toward effectively addressing them. Once we become aware of these external expectations, we can start to question and critically assess them. Understanding that many of these pressures do not accurately reflect our true worth or abilities allows us to approach personal growth and self-acceptance more consciously. Engaging in conversations about these unrealistic societal norms can help teens, young adults, parents, and educators shift their perspectives and nurture a healthier mindset (BetterHelp Editorial Team, 2025).

Once we identify these influences, we can deliberately choose to resist succumbing to them. It's vital to develop strategies for resistance, which serve as essential tools in maintaining self-acceptance and authenticity. For instance, creating critical thinking skills and encouraging open dialogue about these norms can empower young people to question and redefine what success and beauty mean to them.

Parents and educators play a fundamental role in shaping the perspectives of young people, guiding them to understand that achieving societal ideals—such as success, wealth, or social status—is not synonymous with personal value or true happiness. They help young people understand the complexities of societal expectations, encouraging them to explore their own values and passions. By encouraging a supportive environment that celebrates individuality, parents and educators can inspire youth to prioritize their own sense of worth and fulfillment over external validation. This guidance is important for helping the younger generation recognize that real contentment often comes from within rather than from conforming to prescribed norms or measuring their self-worth against societal standards. Through open communication, mentorship, and positive reinforcement, they can cultivate resilience and self-awareness in youth, ultimately empowering them to pursue authentic paths that resonate with their unique identities.

Developing personalized definitions of success and beauty is another key aspect of this journey toward self-acceptance. Success doesn't have to be tied to societal measures such as high-paying jobs or social status. Instead, it can be about achieving personal goals, finding joy in hobbies, or nurturing meaningful relationships. Similarly, redefining beauty to include diverse body types and expressions can significantly enhance self-esteem. The shift from external validation to internal satisfaction supports healthier self-perception and acceptance.

Building confidence through these new definitions is an ongoing process. Focusing on personal strengths and celebrating small achievements allows individuals to create a sense of pride and satisfaction within themselves. Empowering oneself with positive affirmations and surrounding oneself with supportive influences can further reinforce this mindset. It's about reinforcing the notion that self-worth is inherent and not contingent on meeting external criteria.

Community support is vital in helping individuals feel less alone in their struggles. Connecting with like-minded peers, mentors, or support groups provides reassurance and shared experiences. It ensures an environment where individuals can express themselves freely without fear of judgment, thus enhancing a sense of belonging. Such communities can serve as safe spaces for exchanging ideas, sharing challenges, and celebrating achievements together.

Imagine someone moving to a new city, excited about the fresh start but feeling a little lost and alone at first. They don't know anyone yet, and the unfamiliar surroundings make it hard to feel connected. However, they then decide to join a local group for newcomers or a professional network. Suddenly, they start meeting people who understand what they're going through—folks who've been in their shoes and can offer advice or just lend an ear.

As they chat with others, they begin to feel at ease, knowing they're not alone in navigating this new chapter. The group becomes a safe space where they can share their challenges, celebrate small wins, and learn from each other. Over time, these new friendships help them feel like they truly belong, giving them the support and confidence they need to thrive in their new city.

BODY POSITIVITY TECHNIQUES

In today's society, the idea of body positivity has emerged as a powerful movement that encourages individuals to appreciate all body types and experiences. Body positivity is about recognizing the beauty within diversity, an idea that challenges the long-held societal standards of beauty. Recognizing this truth is crucial for individuals seeking self-acceptance in a world dominated by persistent media messages. Promoting body positivity helps individuals appreciate their uniqueness, encouraging them to value themselves in a more holistic way rather than conforming to a narrow ideal.

One effective way to encourage self-love and a healthy body image is by incorporating daily rituals that celebrate one's body. These rituals can be simple yet meaningful practices that encourage self-appreciation. Engaging in activities such as painting, practicing Tai Chi, or reflecting on personal goals and milestones can strengthen a healthy self-perception. For instance, starting the day with a gratitude exercise focused on the body, like acknowledging the strength in one's legs or the warmth of a smile, can shift the focus from perceived flaws to appreciation for what the body enables one to do. Practicing such rituals consistently creates a nurturing relationship with oneself and bolsters self-esteem over time.

Building on this foundation of self-love, another important step toward encouraging self-acceptance involves understanding and identifying triggers for negative body image. Awareness of these triggers allows individuals to proactively manage their responses and develop coping strategies. As we discussed in the previous chapter, triggers could range from certain social media accounts to particular activities that prompt self-comparison or dissatisfaction. Identifying these triggers allows individuals to either reduce their exposure to them or address them with a more critical perspective. Implementing changes, like curating a healthier digital environment or engaging in supportive communities, fosters resilience and diminishes the impacts of these negative influences (*How Can We Protect*, n.d.).

Additionally, embracing the idea that beauty is subjective is pivotal in reinforcing self-worth. Challenging the conventional ideals promoted by media and advertising allows individuals to redefine beauty in more inclusive and personal terms. Beauty extends beyond physical appearance to include qualities such as kindness, intelligence, and creativity. Emphasizing inner attributes alongside outer ones broadens the scope of beauty and empowers individuals to see themselves as valuable regardless of external standards (*Why Body Positivity Is Important*, 2024).

We need to shift the focus from appearance to inner qualities, such as kindness, creativity, and strength, which nurture a deeper, more sustainable sense of self-worth. For example, instead of fixating on how we look in a mirror, we can celebrate how we show kindness to a friend in need or how our creativity helps solve a problem at work. While appearance can change, inner qualities remain constant, allowing us to appreciate ourselves for who we truly are. Valuing kindness helps us recognize our impact on others, creativity encourages self-expression, and strength builds resilience in the face of challenges. This shift not only boosts self-love and confidence but also strengthens our relationships by encouraging us to appreciate others' inner qualities as well.

Body positivity is a powerful experience that enables individuals to celebrate their individuality and redefine conventional standards of beauty. It encourages self-love through daily rituals, builds resilience against societal pressures, and celebrates the diversity of human experiences. Beyond challenging narrow beauty standards, body positivity advocates for representation, inclusivity, and open conversations about self-worth and mental health. By valuing our bodies for their strengths and embracing uniqueness, we challenge societal standards and inspire others.

CELEBRATING INDIVIDUALITY

Embracing your unique qualities is more than just a personal transformation—it's a powerful journey that can significantly enrich your life. When you begin to recognize and accept the traits that define you, you free yourself from the pressure of comparison and open the door to greater confidence, self-esteem, and a deep sense of identity. This journey isn't just about acknowledging who you are but also about celebrating the distinct qualities that make you uniquely you. In doing so, you lay the foundation for a more authentic, fulfilling life.

Recognizing Your True Self

Embracing your distinct qualities can significantly enhance your life experience. The first essential step in this journey is recognizing the traits that define who you are. By acknowledging these personal qualities, you grant yourself the permission to value your individuality, free from the pressure of comparison. This act of self-acceptance sparks confidence and strengthens self-esteem, laying the foundation of a resilient, unshakable identity.

STEPS TO EMBRACE YOUR UNIQUENESS

1. **Identify your distinct characteristics:** Begin by identifying the specific characteristics that make you unique. This involves introspection and reflection, allowing you to see the traits that have shaped you into the person you are today. When you understand these qualities, you can begin to appreciate the true essence of yourself.

2. **Challenge yourself to explore new experiences:** Stepping outside your comfort zone is vital for growth. Pursue new experiences to uncover hidden talents and expand your understanding of what resonates with you. Whether it's taking up a new hobby, such as learning an instrument, or trying a different form of exercise, every new venture can offer valuable insights into your capabilities and interests.

3. **Engage in creative expression:** Creative pursuits offer an excellent outlet for embracing individuality. Activities such as painting, writing, or music enable you to express your inner thoughts and emotions. These artistic forms not only serve as a means of self-expression but also allow you to project your unique identity to others, reinforcing your sense of authenticity.

Celebrating Your Unique Features

Celebrating your uniqueness means appreciating both your intrinsic beauty and distinctive physical traits. It's about seeing yourself in a deeper light beyond conventional standards of beauty. Recognizing and accepting these traits nurtures a compassionate view of yourself, strengthening your self-image. By embracing your uniqueness, you begin to appreciate that what might be perceived as imperfections are actually vital parts of what makes you distinctly beautiful.

GUIDELINES FOR EMBRACING YOUR UNIQUENESS

1. **Identify personal interests and passions:** Start by reflecting on activities and subjects that hold your attention. What are the things you feel most passionate about? These interests often point to deeper aspects of your authentic self and can guide you toward experiences that offer satisfaction and purpose.

2. **Use creative expression as a tool for discovery:** Creative outlets, such as drawing, sculpting, or dance, allow you to explore and communicate your identity. There is no right or wrong when it comes to creativity—only personal expression. Experimenting with various forms of art can unlock hidden talents and deepen your connection with yourself.

3. **Refine and nurture your unique abilities:** Take time to develop the strengths that set you apart from others. Reflect on the skills where you feel most confident, and invest in refining them. These abilities can lead to personal fulfillment and success in various

areas of life. Celebrating even the smallest achievements reinforces the value of your individuality and encourages continual growth.

Living Authentically

Celebrating your individuality goes beyond personal introspection and joy—it encompasses the way you live your life and engage with others. Living genuinely involves aligning your actions with your fundamental values and beliefs. This genuineness builds genuine connections with those around you and attracts relationships that uplift and support your authentic self.

As you grow more confident in who you are, you will naturally attract individuals who appreciate and honor your distinctiveness. Being in the company of such people fortifies your journey toward self-acceptance and establishes a supportive atmosphere for continual personal development.

Valuing your unique characteristics is a deeply fulfilling endeavor that not only boosts your self-esteem but also opens doors for advancement and satisfaction. By recognizing and nurturing your individuality, you set out on a journey that leads to a more genuine existence. Surround yourself with those who champion your pathway, and remain receptive to unveiling new aspects of yourself along the journey. As you persist in acknowledging who you truly are, you build an unwavering confidence that shines through every facet of your life.

PRACTICING SELF-COMPASSION

Self-compassion is essential for our emotional well-being and learning to accept ourselves as we are. It's about treating yourself with the same care and kindness you'd offer a good friend, especially when life gets tough. Rather than falling into the trap of harsh self-criticism, self-compassion encourages you to approach your struggles with patience, understanding, and empathy. By adopting this mindset, you can nurture your mental health, build resilience, and grow a stronger sense of self-worth.

Self-compassion isn't just about being kind to yourself when things go wrong—it's about forming habits that help you recognize and embrace your full humanity, with all its strengths and imperfections. It's a powerful way to counter negative thoughts, boost your self-esteem, and develop a healthier, more positive self-image. Below are some practical steps you can take to bring more self-compassion into your daily routine, helping you grow emotionally and deepen your self-love.

Positive Affirmations

Positive affirmations serve as powerful tools for reshaping your self-talk. Create a list of affirmations that resonate with you and reflect your strengths, values, and personal growth. These affirmations serve as reminders of your inherent worth, helping you stay anchored in a positive self-image.

Make a habit of repeating these affirmations throughout the day, particularly during moments of self-doubt or when facing challenges. For example, say to yourself, "I am deserving of love and respect," or "I am capable of overcoming obstacles, and each setback is a lesson in resilience." Over time, these affirmations will help shift your internal narrative, encouraging a mindset of self-empowerment and compassion.

POSITIVE AFFIRMATIONS

Here are 15 powerful affirmations to elevate your mindset and transform your inner dialogue.

1. I am deserving of love, achievement, and joy.
2. I possess the strength to accomplish any goal I pursue.
3. I have faith in my capacity to make decisions that serve my best interests.
4. Each day, I cultivate greater strength and resilience.
5. I release my fears and welcome self-assurance.
6. I take charge of my emotions and thought patterns.
7. I am worthy of all the blessings that come my way.
8. I consciously choose to dismiss negativity and concentrate on the positive.

9. I recognize my potential and have confidence in my ability to fulfill my dreams.
10. I am sufficient just as I am.
11. I embrace my unique journey and honor my individuality.
12. I am committed to nurturing my happiness and well-being.
13. I attract positive energy and inspiring opportunities.
14. I learn from challenges and use them as stepping stones for growth.
15. I celebrate my progress and acknowledge my achievements, no matter how small.

Self-Kindness Practices

Self-kindness is about treating yourself with the same care and understanding you would offer to a friend. One of the best ways to practice self-kindness is by incorporating activities into your daily routine that bring you joy, relaxation, and peace. Whether it's reading a book, taking a nature walk, practicing a hobby, or simply listening to your favorite music, prioritize moments that recharge your emotional energy.

Self-kindness also means accepting your imperfections and mistakes without harsh judgment. It's vital to recognize that being human involves ups and downs, and no one is immune to mistakes. Instead of focusing on failures, practice gentle self-talk and forgiveness. This helps build resilience and strengthens your capacity to show up for yourself with love and understanding, even in difficult times.

Gratitude Practice

Gratitude can be a powerful tool for cultivating a positive mindset. At the end of each day, take a moment to reflect on three things you're grateful for. These don't have to be monumental events; small things, like a warm cup of tea, a kind interaction, or a moment of peace, count too. Focusing on gratitude helps reframe your perspective, encouraging you to view life through a lens of appreciation instead of scarcity or self-criticism.

Over time, practicing gratitude builds a habit of noticing the positives in your life, even on tough days. It encourages a more compassionate perspective of yourself and your circumstances, reminding you that you are supported and cared for by the world around you, as well as by yourself.

Here are a few different things you can do to encourage gratitude:

- **Gratitude jar:** Keep a jar where you write down things you're grateful for and add a note every time something positive happens. Revisit the jar when you need a mood boost.
- **Daily gratitude journaling:** Write down three to five things you're grateful for each day. Focus on both big and small moments.
- **Gratitude letters:** Write a letter to someone who has made a positive impact on your life. Express your thanks and appreciation for their influence.
- **Gratitude sharing:** Share something you're grateful for with a friend or family member each day. It strengthens your connection and reinforces positive thinking.

GRATITUDE LETTER ACTIVITY

Think of someone in your life who has made a difference—maybe a friend who always has your back, a teacher who believed in you, a family member who supports you, or even someone who showed you kindness when you needed it most.

Now, write them a letter to express your gratitude. Here are some things you can include:

- Start with a warm hello and let them know why you're writing.
- Mention a specific moment when they helped, encouraged, or inspired you.

- Describe how their actions impacted you:
    - ☐ Did they make your day better?
    - ☐ Boost your confidence?
    - ☐ Help you through a tough time?
- Let them know what they mean to you and why you're grateful to have them in your life.
- Close with appreciation and a kind message. You can wish them well, offer to return the favor, or simply say how much you value them.

_____

_____

_____

_____

_____

_____

_____

_____

_____

CHAPTER 5: CULTIVATING SELF-ACCEPTANCE

_____

_____

_____

_____

_____

_____

_____

_____

_____

_____

_____

_____

_____

_____

_____

Self-Compassion Breaks

Throughout the day, take intentional breaks to check in with yourself. These "self-compassion breaks" are moments where you pause, take a deep breath, and assess how you're feeling. During these moments, acknowledge any emotional discomfort without judgment. Instead of pushing through it or criticizing yourself for feeling upset, treat yourself with compassion. Remind yourself that it's okay to experience difficulties and that you don't have to be perfect to be worthy of love and care.

These breaks can be as simple as stepping outside for fresh air, taking a short walk, or practicing deep breathing exercises. Over time, these moments help create a habit of self-care that can make it easier to manage stress and emotional discomfort.

Setting Boundaries With Compassion

Part of practicing self-compassion involves setting healthy boundaries to protect your emotional well-being. This means recognizing when you need to say no or limit your involvement in situations that drain your energy. Setting boundaries isn't about being selfish; it's about acknowledging that your well-being matters and that you deserve to have space to recharge.

When you communicate your boundaries, do so with kindness and clarity. This allows you to take care of your own needs while also respecting others' expectations. Practicing boundary-setting with compassion encourages healthier relationships, both with yourself and others. This will be further discussed in Chapter 6.

Support System and Connection

Building a strong support system, including friends, family, or mentors, is another important aspect of self-compassion. It's vital to surround yourself with people who uplift you, validate your feelings, and encourage your growth. Engaging with others helps to remind you that you are not alone in your experiences, and it provides opportunities to share vulnerabilities and offer support in return.

Make a habit of reaching out to your support system, whether it's for advice, comfort, or simply a friendly chat. Healthy connections remind you that being kind to yourself doesn't mean doing everything alone—it's about embracing community and allowing yourself to be supported.

Incorporating these practices into your routine isn't about achieving perfection; it's about creating a compassionate and nurturing relationship with yourself. The more you commit to these small steps, the more you'll notice a shift in how you perceive and treat yourself. Through patience, self-compassion becomes a natural response, equipping you with the emotional strength and serenity needed to handle the challenges and triumphs of life. This approach encourages a sense of inner calm and acceptance, empowering you to approach life's challenges with gentleness and confidence.

Having explored the impact of societal expectations, it's time to look into the influence of peer pressure on our journey toward self-acceptance. The dynamics of peer relationships often shape our choices, self-image, and boundaries, making it vital to understand how these interactions affect our sense of self. Chapter 6, "Navigating Peer Pressure" provides actionable strategies for effective communication, building assertiveness, and fostering positive relationships. It also addresses how to recognize and manage negative influences, empowering you to create a supportive social environment that aligns with your values and promotes authentic growth.

KEY TAKEAWAYS

- Embracing self-acceptance means reflecting on how societal expectations shape how we see ourselves, often pushing us to conform to narrow ideas of beauty, success, and worth.

- Breaking free from societal pressures involves recognizing and questioning these unrealistic standards so we can prioritize being true to ourselves instead of seeking outside approval.

- Parents and educators are key in helping young people understand their worth, guiding them to define success and beauty on their own terms rather than by society's standards.

- Defining success and beauty for ourselves helps build self-acceptance and brings a sense of inner satisfaction, focusing on what really matters—personal goals and meaningful connections.

- Building confidence through positive affirmations, recognizing our strengths, and celebrating our wins can reinforce the belief that our worth is inherent.

- Support from a community—whether it's friends, peers, or mentors—provides comfort, a sense of belonging, and shared experiences that help strengthen self-acceptance.

- Embracing body positivity encourages us to love our uniqueness, challenge traditional beauty norms, and remember that beauty is different for everyone.

- Practicing self-compassion means treating ourselves kindly in tough times, setting healthy boundaries, and surrounding ourselves with a supportive circle to nurture our emotional well-being.

CHAPTER 6

Navigating Peer Pressure

True empowerment arises when we put our values first, letting go of the pressure to conform and allowing our authentic selves to flourish.

Navigating peer pressure is a journey we all face, particularly during the formative years of adolescence and early adulthood. Peer pressure can arise in various settings, from school hallways to online social circles, each presenting unique challenges that test our ability to remain authentic amid external influences. It is a moment when the urge to conform frequently clashes with our core beliefs, rendering the experience of managing these pressures both intricate and essential. Recognizing the subtle ways peer influence affects decision-making and self-identity is key to learning how to handle these situations effectively. Beneath this challenge, however, lies an opportunity for growth and resilience, helping us strengthen our inner voice and sense of self even when surrounded by diverse perspectives and expectations.

STRATEGIES FOR COMMUNICATION

Expressing thoughts and feelings calmly and assertively is important for managing peer pressure. Effective communication skills provide individuals with the ability to share their experiences clearly, preventing conflicts and misunderstandings. In this section, we'll explore various strategies, offering practical guidance for young people, parents, educators, and wellness professionals alike.

Active listening is essential for successful communication. It involves fully engaging with a speaker, and when you actively listen, you're not just hearing words; you're interpreting emotions, intent, and meaning behind those words. This approach helps in crafting a thoughtful response rather than an impulsive reaction. For instance, maintaining eye contact and nodding occasionally shows the speaker that you are invested in the conversation. Providing verbal affirmations like "I see what you mean" or "That makes sense" also reinforces this engagement, creating a space where both parties feel heard and valued (Robinson et al., 2025). We go further into active listening in Chapter 9.

Using "I" statements is another powerful technique that ensures honest communication while reducing blame. Phrases like "I feel concerned when..." allow individuals to share their perspectives without sounding accusatory. This approach promotes a more open and nondefensive conversation, encouraging constructive dialogue. It helps people express how certain actions affect them personally, creating space for empathy and understanding. For instance, instead of saying, "You never listen to me," which might trigger defensiveness, one could say, "I feel unheard when my suggestions aren't taken into account." This simple change in language can significantly improve communication and lead to more meaningful exchanges (Stef, 2023).

Practicing assertiveness is pivotal for maintaining one's beliefs and boundaries while interacting respectfully with others. Being assertive means expressing your needs and desires clearly and confidently without dismissing or infringing on others' rights.

Techniques such as empathy mapping help you understand both your perspective and the emotions, needs, and concerns of others. For example, imagine you need to tell a colleague that their frequent interruptions during meetings make it difficult for you to contribute. Before addressing the issue, you create an empathy map:

- **Think:** What might your colleague believe about their behavior? Perhaps they think their interruptions demonstrate enthusiasm or expertise.
- **Feel:** They may feel unappreciated if they perceive their input isn't valued.
- **Say:** They might express defensiveness if approached too directly.
- **Do:** They might interrupt again without realizing its impact.

Using this empathy map, you can craft a response that acknowledges their intentions while asserting your needs. You might say: "I appreciate your enthusiasm during meetings, but I've noticed that when you interject, it can be challenging for me to share my perspective. I'd like to ensure we both have opportunities to contribute." This method helps you express your feelings while also considering your coworker's thoughts, leading to positive results for everyone involved.

Now, when it comes to ensuring that our messages are accurately interpreted, the significance of nonverbal communication can't be overstated. Body language, facial expressions, and other nonverbal cues can often speak more powerfully than words. Positive gestures, such as maintaining an open posture, steady eye contact, and a warm smile, can strengthen the message and help foster trust. On the other hand, negative signals like crossed arms, avoiding eye contact, or aggressive movements can undermine what we're trying to convey and create confusion. For example, if someone says they're open to feedback but shows closed-off body language, it can come across as disingenuous. Being aware of and managing these nonverbal cues can significantly improve communication and contribute to stronger, more positive relationships (Stef, 2023).

Applying these techniques in everyday conversations empowers individuals to handle peer pressure more effectively. Whether it's dealing with friends, family, or educators, employing active listening, using "I" statements, practicing assertiveness, and mastering nonverbal communication can create pathways for resolving misunderstandings and promoting deeper connections. These skills are vital in resisting negative influences and for building meaningful, supportive relationships that respect each individual's ideas and perspectives.

BUILDING ASSERTIVENESS

The ability to articulate emotions and advocate for one's needs is essential for effectively managing peer influence. Recognizing individual rights within social contexts is the first step toward this empowerment. Understanding that everyone has the right to express their own thoughts and emotions without being judged or belittled can be tremendously liberating. This sense of entitlement to one's own feelings helps individuals stand firm in their identities and maintain confidence when faced with conflicting opinions from peers.

Understanding Rights in Social Contexts

A vital part of understanding your rights involves identifying where they intersect with others. Social contexts often blur these lines, making it challenging to discern when to assert oneself. By recognizing that everyone's perspectives hold value but are not inherently superior, people can engage in interactions without feeling diminished. It's important, then, to appreciate the balance between standing up for oneself and listening to others, as mutual respect encourages an environment where all voices can be heard.

The Role of Role-Playing

Role-playing scenarios present practical ways to rehearse handling peer pressure and asserting your personal needs. Simulating real-life encounters in a controlled setting allows you to gain valuable experience and reduce anxiety associated with these situations. For instance, practicing how to decline certain requests or articulate personal preferences can make these decisions feel less intimidating in real-life scenarios. Role-play provides an opportunity to experiment with different responses, helping individuals discover what feels most authentic and effective for them. Imagine a scenario where a group of friends pressures someone to attend a party they're uncomfortable with. In a role-playing exercise, the individual practices responding by confidently saying, "Thanks for inviting me, but I'm going to sit this one out." They might also rehearse redirecting the conversation by suggesting an alternative activity, such as, "How about we hang out another time and do something we all enjoy?" Practicing this scenario allows them to experiment with their tone, body language, and choice of words, ultimately building the confidence to authentically assert their needs when confronted with similar pressures in real life.

Establishing Personal Boundaries

Deliberately establishing personal boundaries is vital for safeguarding oneself against harmful influences. These boundaries serve as a guide for what behaviors and interactions are acceptable, ensuring that individuals do not compromise their self-worth or independence. Setting boundaries involves recognizing your limits and communicating them clearly to others. For instance, if a friend suggests engaging in activities that conflict with personal values, expressing discomfort and stating clear boundaries reinforces self-worth and demonstrates commitment to one's principles. Establishing boundaries requires ongoing reflection and adaptation. As life circumstances change, so too might the necessity of certain limits. Regularly revisiting and reassessing these boundaries ensures they continue to serve your mental well-being. If maintained effectively, they become a powerful tool for nurturing autonomy and promoting a balanced life. Practicing boundary-setting allows individuals to carve out spaces where they feel safe and respected, which is a fundamental component of self-care and mental health.

Communicating Boundaries Effectively

For example, boundaries might involve setting limits on how much time you're willing to give to others or defining when you need personal space. Phrases like "I need some time for myself" or "I'm unable to help with that right now, but thanks for asking" can be clear ways to express those boundaries. Boundaries could also involve limiting emotional or financial involvement in relationships, such as saying, "I'm not comfortable discussing this topic" or "I've reached my limit in supporting you financially." Boundaries should be set when you feel your needs are being overlooked or when others' behaviors begin to encroach on your personal space, energy, or resources. For instance, if you notice a friend repeatedly asking for favors or emotional support without reciprocating, it's important to set a boundary. You might say, "I've noticed I've been giving a lot of time and energy to this relationship, and I need a more balanced dynamic." Similarly, if a friend's behavior is starting to make you uncomfortable, you could assert, "I need to set a limit here because I feel like I'm being taken advantage of." Identifying when these patterns emerge and asserting boundaries at the right moments is essential to maintaining healthy, respectful relationships while protecting your well-being.

Handling Conflict Constructively

In a society where expectations can challenge individuality, it's important to handle conflicts while staying true to your beliefs. Handling disagreement constructively is another skill that enhances critical thinking and appreciation for diverse opinions. Approaching conflicts with an open mind encourages dialogue rather than confrontation. This entails actively listening to opposing views and seeking to understand rather than simply rebutting. Appreciating the differing perspectives presented in disagreements ensures a collaborative environment where solutions can arise through mutual respect.

Developing Communication Skills

Developing effective communication and conflict resolution skills is vital for promoting healthy relationships and maintaining personal well-being.

This may involve using techniques such as active listening and paraphrasing to ensure that both parties feel heard and understood. It's also essential to address conflicts with a calm demeanor, focusing on the issue rather than personalizing the disagreement. This approach helps minimize emotional escalation and encourages greater awareness of personal biases and assumptions that might shape your perspective.

The Benefits of Constructive Conflict Resolution

Constructive conflict resolution strengthens interpersonal skills and fosters stronger relationships over time. It encourages individuals to embrace diversity, recognizing that varied experiences and beliefs contribute to a more holistic understanding of the world. Successfully managing these discussions strengthens one's ability to advocate for personal beliefs while honoring the rights of others.

Supporting Self-Awareness and Resilience

Creating an environment that promotes self-awareness and resilience is fundamental to supporting these strategies. Developing a strong sense of self-awareness allows individuals to identify personal triggers and areas where they might need assertiveness reinforcement. Engaging in therapeutic activities can uncover underlying motivations and fears that hinder assertiveness, paving the way for clearer communication and self-advocacy. Resilience works hand in hand with assertiveness, providing individuals with the emotional strength to withstand external pressures. Developing resilience means learning from challenges and seeing them as opportunities for growth rather than viewing them as failures. By focusing on building inner strength, individuals become better equipped to stand firm against outside influences, which, in turn, boosts their confidence in asserting themselves.

IDENTIFYING POSITIVE RELATIONSHIPS

As we navigate peer pressure and life's challenges, it's essential to recognize and invest in relationships that promote personal growth. Healthy friendships are an essential part of emotional well-being, built on support, mutual respect, and understanding. These friendships provide a safe space for open expression, free from judgment, while creating a sense of belonging and validation. In this section, we'll explore the core elements of healthy friendships and how they contribute to both individual growth and community well-being.

The Role of Healthy Friendships in Personal Growth

Friendships are not just social connections; they are vital to personal development and emotional health. Supportive friends encourage one another's goals, celebrate achievements, and provide comfort during challenging times. These friendships offer a sounding board for feedback, helping individuals build resilience and develop positive coping strategies. For instance, when doubt creeps in, a friend who listens and encourages you can significantly alter how you perceive challenges, making them feel more manageable.

A healthy friendship thrives on mutual respect and genuine understanding. Respect involves acknowledging each other's boundaries, even when perspectives differ. It requires active listening and valuing the other person's feelings and experiences. In healthy friendships, disagreements are resolved with empathy and openness, strengthening the bond between friends. This mutual respect creates an environment where diverse opinions are valued and understood.

Understanding goes beyond active listening—it involves being in tune with a friend's emotions and perspectives. This empathy allows friends to adjust their behavior to support one another, helping reduce stress and enhance emotional well-being. Building understanding in friendships promotes a supportive environment and reduces conflict.

Positive Characteristics of a Healthy Friendship

Friendships play a vital role in our lives, offering emotional support and encouraging a sense of belonging. A healthy friendship is characterized by several key traits that nurture trust, respect, and growth. These characteristics ensure that the bond between friends remains strong and meaningful over time.

- **Support:** A healthy friendship is built on mutual support, where friends encourage each other's goals and celebrate achievements without jealousy or resentment.

- **Trust:** Trust is foundational in any strong friendship. Both friends feel safe being open and honest with each other, knowing that their thoughts and feelings will be respected.

- **Respect:** In a healthy friendship, respect for each other's boundaries, opinions, and choices is essential. Disagreements are handled with empathy and understanding, allowing both people to feel heard.

- **Empathy:** Friends in a healthy relationship try to understand each other's emotions and perspectives, offering comfort and compassion when needed.

- **Communication:** Open and clear communication helps resolve misunderstandings and strengthens the bond. Healthy friends share their feelings and listen actively.

- **Fun and enjoyment:** A key trait of a healthy friendship is enjoying each other's company. Whether it's sharing a laugh or participating in activities together, a sense of joy is always present.

- **Mutual growth:** In a healthy friendship, both friends encourage each other's personal development and growth, providing constructive feedback and helping each other become better versions of themselves.

These various traits are discussed throughout the chapters of this book and will guide you in becoming an exceptional friend and assist you in discovering tranquility in your relationships.

Assessing and Maintaining Healthy Friendships

Regularly reflecting on your relationships is an essential step in maintaining healthy friendships. Not all connections bring positivity into your life. Toxic friendships can leave you feeling drained, anxious, or insecure. Assessing the influence of each connection allows you to identify which friendships encourage your development and which may impede it. If a relationship consistently brings negativity, it may be time to set boundaries or distance yourself to protect your well-being.

Surrounding yourself with supportive, optimistic friends creates an environment conducive to personal growth. Healthy relationships inspire confidence and self-worth, whereas toxic ones erode them. Reflecting on your friendships ensures you create space for connections that uplift and encourage, enhancing your emotional resilience.

Building a Supportive Network

Building a supportive network means not only maintaining current friendships but also finding new connections that match your values and goals. A strong network gives you a sense of belonging and boosts self-acceptance. Joining activities that reflect your interests—like clubs, volunteering, or community events—helps you meet people with similar values. These shared experiences create a strong foundation for lasting friendships.

Deepening friendships come from spending meaningful time together. Whether it's attending an event or having a simple conversation, these moments build trust and strengthen the bond. Shared memories help create a lasting, resilient connection.

Balancing Online and In-Person Connections

Technology makes it easy to stay connected, but it shouldn't replace face-to-face interactions. Meeting in person creates stronger, more genuine connections, fostering closeness and better understanding. While digital communication helps keep in touch, in-person time deepens friendships in ways online chats can't match. Finding a balance between digital and in-person communication is key to building lasting, meaningful friendships.

Nurturing and maintaining healthy friendships is essential for both personal growth and emotional well-being. These relationships offer unmatched support, helping individuals remain resilient through life's challenges. By investing time and energy into building and nurturing these connections, we encourage emotional fulfillment and lasting happiness.

DEALING WITH NEGATIVE INFLUENCES

Facing the challenges of peer pressure can be overwhelming, particularly for teenagers and young adults who are at a crucial stage in shaping their identities. One fundamental aspect of managing these influences is identifying toxic behaviors within friendships. Recognizing these patterns is essential as they often subtly undermine an individual's well-being. Toxic behaviors may manifest as consistent negativity, manipulation, or a lack of support, leaving one feeling drained or distressed after interactions. It is important to pay attention to how you feel after spending time with certain people. If someone consistently makes you feel worse rather than better, this might indicate that the relationship is detrimental.

Recognizing Toxic Behaviors

Toxic behaviors can be disruptive and emotionally draining, often going unnoticed until they've already had a significant impact. These behaviors can take many forms, from negativity to manipulation, and can slowly erode the quality of relationships, whether at home, in your community, or at work.

SIGNS OF TOXIC BEHAVIORS

Consistent negativity

- ☐ A constant focus on what's wrong or what could go wrong rather than seeking solutions or celebrating positives.
- ☐ Repeated complaints about life or others without any intention to improve or resolve the situation.

☐ This kind of negativity can leave you feeling drained, as it often doesn't allow space for growth, optimism, or progress.

Manipulation

☐ Subtle or overt efforts to control or guilt-trip others into doing things they may not want to do.

☐ Emotional manipulation through gaslighting (making others doubt their reality or perception) or using someone's vulnerabilities to create dependency.

☐ Manipulative behaviors often aim to shift the power dynamic, leaving you second-guessing your decisions and making you feel helpless or confused.

Lack of support

☐ A consistent pattern of withdrawing support or empathy when it's most needed, leaving you to feel alone, unimportant, or unappreciated.

☐ Indifference to your successes, struggles, or emotional needs, often masking this as indifference or "tough love."

Impact of Negative Relationships

The impact of such negative relationships on emotional health can be harmful. They can cause insecurity, anxiety, or feelings of worthlessness. For instance, a friend who belittles your achievements or constantly questions your choices can erode your self-esteem over time. This erosion affects not just personal happiness but also the ability to make proactive life choices. Once these toxic influences are identified, steps can be taken to minimize their impact, which leads us to discuss the importance of creating distance from harmful relationships.

CREATING DISTANCE FROM HARMFUL RELATIONSHIPS

This process of distancing doesn't necessarily mean cutting ties abruptly unless absolutely necessary. Instead, it involves setting boundaries that prioritize your mental and emotional health. Gently reducing contact or interacting in group settings rather than one-on-one helps protect your well-being while allowing you to evaluate the future of the friendship. This distance provides space for personal growth and emotional recovery, enabling you to refocus on the positive aspects of life. As you create this distance, you'll find room to breathe, reflect, and invest time in activities and relationships that fuel positivity.

IMPORTANCE OF OPEN COMMUNICATION

A significant step toward improving any relationship affected by negative peer influence is open communication. Addressing concerns directly with friends can lead to clarity and mutual understanding. While it may seem daunting, having honest conversations about what upsets you creates opportunities for change and accountability. Expressing how specific actions or words impact you gives your friends an opportunity to adjust their behavior, promoting a healthier connection. Open dialogue also acts as a litmus test, helping you determine whether the relationship is worth nurturing or requires re-evaluation.

STRENGTHENING FRIENDSHIPS THROUGH COMMUNICATION

Often, communicating your concerns will strengthen your friendships. When approached with respect and empathy, these conversations can result in deeper bonds and greater emotional support. On the other hand, if the response is dismissive or defensive, it may confirm the need to free yourself from these relationships. Remember, true friends will appreciate you voicing your feelings and be willing to work toward mutual respect and understanding. The power of transparency and genuine communication cannot be overstated in creating secure and supportive social circles.

SEEKING HEALTHIER SOCIAL INTERACTIONS

In moving away from negative influences, it's equally important to seek out healthier social interactions. Finding environments where positivity thrives can introduce new perspectives and sources of encouragement. Embracing diversity in your social network enhances resilience by providing a wide array of experiences and insights. Healthy friendships contribute significantly to one's emotional well-being by offering companionship, reassurance, and constructive feedback. Being around supportive peers helps shift focus from negative pressures to the numerous possibilities that come with positive relationships. Additionally, these connections serve as valuable resources during challenging times, supplying comfort and guidance when needed.

MAKING DELIBERATE CHOICES ABOUT SOCIAL CIRCLES

Understanding that handling peer pressure involves making deliberate choices about whom you associate with is important. Choosing to be around individuals who inspire and support you while distancing yourself from those who drain your energy builds meaningful relationships that enhance your personal development and satisfaction. This process requires ongoing self-examination to identify friendships that contribute positively to your growth and those that may hinder it. Regularly assessing your social networks ensures they align with your aspirations and principles, setting the stage for a more genuine and rewarding life.

PRIORITIZING YOUR VALUES

Remember, peer pressure is not about shying away from difficult situations; rather, it is about celebrating your uniqueness and making decisions that reflect your core principles. Embracing who you are allows you to withstand external expectations and stand firm in your beliefs. In a world filled with influences, it is essential to prioritize your values, ensuring that every choice you make resonates with your true self. This intentional approach empowers you to confront challenges head-on while remaining authentic.

STEPS TO SETTING BOUNDARIES WITH FRIENDS

Identify the Boundaries You Need

Before setting boundaries, take time to reflect on what is making you uncomfortable or draining your energy. Boundaries can relate to time, emotions, communication, or behavior.

Ask Yourself:

- What specific behaviors make me feel uncomfortable, disrespected, or overwhelmed?
- In what ways does this friendship feel unbalanced?
- Have I felt obligated to say "yes" when I really wanted to say "no"?
- Do I feel drained or disrespected after spending time with this person?

Common Types of Boundaries in Friendships:

- **Time boundaries:** limiting how much time you spend with someone so you have space for yourself
- **Emotional boundaries:** not taking on all of their problems or feeling responsible for their emotions
- **Communication boundaries:** choosing when and how often to engage in conversations, especially about heavy or negative topics
- **Behavioral boundaries:** addressing actions that make you uncomfortable, such as gossiping, controlling behavior, or constant criticism

Example Situations and Boundaries

- **Situation:** Your friend constantly calls late at night, disrupting your sleep.
- **Boundary:** "I need to be in bed by 10 p.m., so I won't be answering calls after that time."

- **Situation:** Your friend vents about their problems but never asks how you're doing.
- **Boundary:** "I care about you, but I also need space to share my thoughts. Can we make our conversations more balanced?"

- **Situation:** Your friend pressures you into activities that you don't enjoy.
- **Boundary:** "I appreciate the invite, but I'm not comfortable doing that. Let's find something we both enjoy."

Communicate Your Boundaries Clearly

Once you've identified what boundaries you need, communicate them with honesty and confidence. Don't assume your friend knows they're crossing a line—be clear and direct.

HOW TO COMMUNICATE BOUNDARIES EFFECTIVELY

- Be assertive, not aggressive. Use calm and respectful language.
- Use "I" statements to express your needs without blaming them.

   Example: Instead of saying, "You never listen to me," say, "I feel unheard when our conversations only focus on your concerns."

- Be specific about what you need.

   Example: "I need more personal time on weekends, so I won't always be available to hang out."

What Not to Do:

- Don't apologize for setting boundaries ("Sorry, but I just need space").
- Don't make your boundaries sound optional ("I kind of feel like I need space...").
- Don't let guilt override your needs.

Stand Firm and Enforce Your Boundaries

It's common for people to test boundaries, especially if they're used to having unrestricted access to your time and energy. If a friend ignores your boundary, it's important to reinforce it consistently.

WHAT TO DO IF THEY PUSH BACK

- **If they ignore your boundary:**
  Calmly remind them: "I mentioned that I can't talk late at night. Let's catch up earlier in the day instead."
- **If they make you feel guilty:**
  Stay firm: "I understand that you're upset, but I need to take care of my own well-being too."
- **If they try to manipulate you:**
  Recognize toxic behavior and consider distancing yourself.

Red Flags That Indicate a Lack of Respect for Boundaries:

- They try to guilt-trip you into doing things you don't want to do.
- They act entitled to your time and energy.
- They repeatedly ignore your requests, even after multiple reminders.
- They make you feel bad for prioritizing yourself.

People who truly respect and value your friendship will honor your boundaries, even if they take time to adjust.

Adjust and Re-Evaluate If Needed

Boundaries aren't set in stone. As your friendship evolves, you may need to adjust your limits. Check in with yourself regularly to see if your needs are being met.

SIGNS YOUR BOUNDARIES NEED ADJUSTING

- You still feel drained or uncomfortable despite setting limits.
- Your friend continues to disregard your needs.
- You feel guilty or anxious about maintaining your boundaries.

What to Do If Your Friend Respects Your Boundaries:

- Acknowledge their effort and appreciation: "I really appreciate you understanding my need for space. It means a lot."
- Be open to compromise if it aligns with your comfort level.

Know When to Walk Away

If a friend continuously disrespects your boundaries and makes you feel unvalued, it may be time to reconsider the friendship. A one-sided friendship that disregards your well-being is not worth maintaining.

WHEN TO END THE FRIENDSHIP

- Your boundaries are repeatedly ignored, even after clear communication.
- The friendship consistently makes you feel drained or anxious.
- They manipulate, guilt-trip, or disrespect you when you enforce your limits.
- You feel like you're walking on eggshells around them.

How to End It Gracefully (If Necessary):

- **Gradually distance yourself:** Reduce time spent with them and disengage from constant contact.
- **Have a direct conversation:** If necessary, let them know why you're stepping back.
- **Go no-contact if needed:** If they are toxic or abusive, cutting ties completely is an option.

Ending a friendship does not reflect poorly on you; it signifies a commitment to self-respect. Establishing boundaries with friends isn't about exclusion; it's about nurturing healthier, more balanced connections. Boundaries safeguard your emotional well-being while promoting relationships grounded in mutual respect. Genuine friendships will endure and thrive through the process of setting limits, while those that falter may indicate underlying issues that need attention. Keep in mind that your responsibility lies in honoring your needs, not in managing how others react to your boundaries.

QUESTIONS TO EVALUATE WHETHER YOUR FRIENDSHIP IS A POSITIVE OR NEGATIVE INFLUENCE ON YOU

Do I feel energized and encouraged by my friend or friend group?
Do I often leave feeling fatigued and disheartened after spending time with my friends?

_____

_____

_____

_____

_____

_____

_____

This question explores the emotional energy of the friendship. Positive friendships should leave you feeling supported, motivated, and uplifted, while negative friendships may cause feelings of exhaustion, discouragement, or emotional depletion. It reveals whether your friend is contributing to your well-being or if the relationship is taking a toll on your mental health.

If you feel drained or discouraged:

- Take note of how you feel after spending time with this friend. Do you leave feeling inspired and valued or exhausted and emotionally depleted?
- If you consistently feel drained, reflect on whether their behavior is negative, critical, or dismissive.
- Consider limiting interactions and spending more time with people who uplift and support you.
- If you want to salvage the friendship, have an honest conversation about how their behavior affects you.

Does this friend encourage my personal growth and success?
Do my friends undermine my goals and dreams?

_____

_____

_____

_____

_____

_____

This question explores your friend's response to your goals and accomplishments. A supportive friendship will encourage you to be ambitious, celebrate your victories, and facilitate your growth. If a friend diminishes your dreams, trivializes your accomplishments, or overlooks your potential, it indicates a harmful or unsupportive relationship that could hinder your personal development.

If they undermine your goals:

- Notice if they dismiss your achievements, minimize your goals, or make you feel foolish for aiming high.
- Ask yourself whether their negativity stems from their own insecurities or jealousy.
- Try sharing your aspirations with other friends who genuinely celebrate your success.
- If the negativity persists, distance yourself and surround yourself with people who genuinely want to see you grow.

How does this friend react when I share my accomplishments or challenges with them?

_____

_____

_____

_____

_____

_____

_____

_____

_____

_____

_____

_____

_____

_____

_____

_____

_____

_____

_____

This question reveals whether your friend is genuinely invested in your well-being. A supportive friend will celebrate your wins with joy and provide comfort or empathy when you face challenges. On the other hand, if your friend reacts with indifference, jealousy, or criticism, it signals that they may not have your best interests at heart and might not be a positive influence in your life.

If they react negatively (jealousy, indifference, or criticism):

- Pay attention to their tone and body language when you share good news.
- If they frequently dismiss or downplay your successes, it may be a sign that they aren't truly happy for you.
- If they make everything about themselves when you express struggles, they might not be emotionally available to support you.
- Consider having a candid discussion about how their reactions make you feel and see if their behavior changes.

Does this friendship contribute positively to my mental and emotional well-being?

_____

_____

_____

_____

_____

_____

This question uncovers the emotional impact the friendship has on your mental health. Friendships should help alleviate stress and foster positive feelings, but if a friendship is constantly a source of tension, anxiety, or emotional strain, it could be harmful to your well-being. It forces you to examine whether the relationship brings peace or if it contributes to unnecessary emotional turmoil.

If no (it causes stress and anxiety):

- Reflect on whether your stress comes from conflicts, criticism, or feeling undervalued.
- If their presence frequently brings you stress rather than joy, it may be time to step away.
- A healthy friendship should bring comfort and security, not emotional exhaustion.
- Set boundaries, limit your interactions, and seek friendships that nurture your well-being.

Do you maintain open, honest communication with your friends?

_____

_____

_____

_____

_____

Effective communication forms the foundation of strong friendships. This question allows you to evaluate whether the relationship is based on shared trust and open conversations. If you find yourself hesitant to discuss significant issues due to anxiety or discomfort, it indicates a lack of sincerity and openness in the friendship, hindering the possibility of a more meaningful and genuine bond.

If no (you feel like you're walking on eggshells):

- Ask yourself why—do they react badly to constructive feedback or serious discussions?
- If you feel like you constantly have to filter your words to avoid upsetting them, this could indicate an unhealthy dynamic.
- A real friend should be open to discussing problems and working through them together.
- If the friendship lacks honest communication, consider addressing the issue directly or evaluating whether this relationship is worth maintaining.

Do I feel valued and respected in this friendship?

_____

_____

_____

_____

_____

This question helps you evaluate whether your feelings, needs, and boundaries are respected in the friendship. Feeling valued and respected is a sign of a healthy relationship, whereas feeling dismissed or unimportant indicates that the friendship may be one-sided or not rooted in mutual respect. A lack of respect often leads to emotional harm and imbalance in the relationship.

If no (you feel dismissed):

- Identify whether your opinions, feelings, or boundaries are regularly ignored.
- If you feel like your presence doesn't matter to them, it may be time to distance yourself.
- Respect is a nonnegotiable part of any meaningful relationship—if it's missing, the friendship may not be serving you.
- Express your concerns and observe their response—do they make an effort to change or continue to dismiss you?

Do I feel like I am the only one putting in effort in this friendship?

_____

_____

_____

_____

_____

_____

_____

Healthy friendships are reciprocal, with both parties contributing to the relationship. If you're always the one reaching out, initiating plans, or supporting your friend without receiving the same level of effort in return, it can feel exhausting and one-sided. This question helps you evaluate whether the friendship is a two-way street or if you're carrying more than your fair share of the emotional labor.

If you feel it is a one-sided friendship:

- Take a break from initiating contact and see if they reach out.
- If you're always the one making plans, checking in, and offering support without receiving the same in return, the friendship may be unbalanced.
- Consider addressing the issue directly with your friend.
- If they don't change or show appreciation for your efforts, redirect your energy toward relationships that value you.

Do you feel like you have to change who you are to fit in with your friend group?

_____

_____

_____

_____

_____

_____

_____

_____

_____

_____

_____

_____

_____

_____

_____

_____

_____

_____

_____

_____

_____

Authenticity is key to genuine friendships. This question reveals whether you feel accepted and free to be your true self around your friend or whether you feel pressured to change your behavior, values, or personality to fit in with their expectations. A good friend should encourage you to embrace who you are, not make you feel like you need to alter yourself to gain their approval.

If you feel like you have to change around your friends:

- Ask yourself why—are they judgmental, critical, or dismissive of certain aspects of your personality?
- Friendships should feel safe and allow you to express yourself without fear.
- If you constantly adjust your personality to fit their expectations, the friendship may not be authentic.
- Seek relationships where you feel accepted for who you truly are.

Does this friend respect my boundaries?

Do they frequently push me to do things I'm uncomfortable with?

_____

_____

_____

_____

_____

_____

Respecting boundaries is essential for any healthy relationship. This question highlights whether your friend acknowledges and respects your personal limits or whether they pressure you into situations where you feel uncomfortable. Friends who respect your boundaries allow you to maintain a sense of safety and trust, while those who overstep them can create feelings of discomfort and resentment.

If they frequently push your limits:

- Firmly reinforce your boundaries and observe their response.
- A true friend will honor your comfort zone, while a toxic one may continue to push or guilt you into situations you don't want to be in.
- If they repeatedly ignore your limits, it's a sign that they do not respect you.
- Limit interactions with people who disregard your needs and personal values.

How does this friend make me feel about myself in the long run—more confident and secure, or more insecure and self-doubting?

_____

_____

_____

_____

_____

_____

This is a reflection on the long-term effects of the friendship on your self-esteem. A positive friendship should help build your confidence and sense of self-worth. If a friend regularly makes you feel insecure, self-doubting, or less than you are, it's a sign that the friendship is unhealthy. Friendships that chip away at your self-esteem can undermine your confidence and hold you back from being your best self.

If they make you insecure:

- Take note of whether their words or actions contribute to feelings of self-doubt.
- If they constantly criticize, compare, or make you feel inadequate, they are likely harming your self-esteem.
- Surround yourself with people who uplift and empower you, not those who make you feel lesser.
- If they are unaware of their impact, consider expressing your feelings and see if they're willing to change.

In the next chapter, we explore mindful breathing techniques, yoga poses for stress relief, and how to incorporate mindfulness into daily life. These practices offer effective tools for managing stress, enhancing emotional well-being, and improving mental clarity. These methods will empower you to tackle life's obstacles with enhanced composure and strength.

KEY TAKEAWAYS

- Dealing with peer pressure is a common challenge in adolescence and early adulthood, as individuals face external influences that challenge their authenticity.

- Effective communication techniques, such as active listening, using "I" statements, and assertiveness, help individuals express their thoughts and needs clearly while managing peer pressure.

- Building assertiveness involves recognizing one's rights and expressing emotions in social situations, empowering individuals to stand up for themselves while respecting others.

- Practicing conflict resolution and valuing diverse viewpoints promotes healthy relationships and encourages constructive discussions rather than confrontations.

- Identifying positive relationships is essential for personal growth; supportive, respectful, and understanding friendships enhance emotional well-being.

- Recognizing toxic behaviors like manipulation and negativity helps individuals assess their friendships and protect their mental health from harmful influences.

- Setting and communicating boundaries is key to maintaining healthy friendships, safeguarding emotional well-being, and ensuring mutual respect.

- Regularly reassessing friendships allows individuals to nurture positive connections and distance themselves from negative influences, creating an environment that supports personal growth and self-acceptance.

BREATHE. RELEASE. RESTORE.

7 DAYS TO EMOTIONAL FREEDOM

You get a FREE 7-day guided video experience
built to help you calm your mind,
reset your energy, and feel lighter every day.

Chapter 7 breaks down the breathing exercises and
yoga moves you'll use throughout your journey.

For a head start, skim Chapter 7 to get the
full overview. Then scan the QR code below
or visit **www.BreatheReleaseRestore.com**
to begin your 7-day reset.

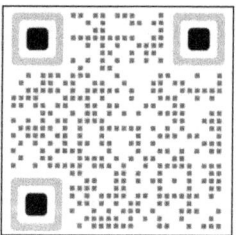

Watch **ONE video per day**, then jump back
into the chapters ahead to lock in what you've
learned with real reflection and practice.

BREATHE. RELEASE. RESTORE.

———

Stress Management Through Mindful Exercises

In the mosaic of life, stress-reduction activities are the vibrant tiles—each one a unique experience that contributes to the masterpiece of emotional balance and inner peace.

Managing stress is essential in today's fast-paced world, and mindfulness can be your most powerful tool. In this chapter, you'll discover practical mindfulness techniques to help you navigate your emotional landscape with greater ease. Let's start with one of the simplest yet most impactful practices: mindful breathing. Breathing isn't just a biological function—it's a direct line to grounding yourself in the present moment. Mastering mindful breathing techniques creates a sense of calm regardless of how chaotic life gets.

MINDFUL BREATHING TECHNIQUES

Breathing is an often-overlooked yet powerful tool in stress management. By tapping into various breathing techniques, you can create a sense of calm and presence, easing stress and anxiety. In this section, we explore several effective breathing practices designed to help you ground yourself in the present moment and help manage stress. These exercises can be performed in various locations; however, it is recommended that you practice these techniques in tranquil, open spaces with minimal auditory distractions.

Deep Diaphragmatic Breathing

Unlike shallow chest breathing, deep diaphragmatic breathing engages the diaphragm, allowing the lungs to fill completely and promoting relaxation. This technique lowers your heart rate, reduces tension, and helps you feel more grounded.

HOW TO PRACTICE

1. Sit comfortably and place one hand on your abdomen.
2. Inhale deeply through your nose, letting your abdomen expand.
3. Exhale slowly, feeling your abdomen contract.
4. Repeat this process, focusing on the slow, deliberate pace of each breath.

Regular practice of deep diaphragmatic breathing enhances body awareness and can lead to a calmer, more centered state, helping you manage anxiety and improve emotional well-being.

Box Breathing

Box breathing is a structured technique that involves equal timing for inhaling, holding, exhaling, and pausing. This method is particularly useful for beginners and can be easily adapted to various situations, like stressful meetings and moments of anxiety.

HOW TO PRACTICE

1. Inhale through your nose for a count of four.
2. Hold your breath at the top for a count of four.
3. Exhale slowly through your mouth for a count of four.
4. Hold your breath out for a final count of four.
5. Repeat the sequence several times.

Imagine you're about to give a presentation, and you're feeling nervous. Instead of letting the anxiety take over, you decide to use box breathing to calm your mind and focus.

You take a moment to sit quietly and start by inhaling deeply through your nose for a count of four. You then hold your breath for a count of four, allowing yourself to feel centered. Slowly, you exhale through your mouth for a count of four, releasing any tension. Finally, you hold your breath out for another count of four.

After repeating this sequence a few times, you notice your heart rate slows, and you feel more grounded. Your mind is clearer, and you're better prepared to face the presentation with a calm and focused mindset. Box breathing has helped you regain control over your stress, turning a potentially overwhelming moment into an opportunity for calm and clarity.

Sighing Breath

An effective method for alleviating accumulated stress in just a few deep breaths.

HOW TO PRACTICE

1. Take a deep breath in through your nose.
2. Exhale with an audible sigh.
3. Repeat three to four times, allowing your body to relax.

Resonant Breathing

This technique helps synchronize breathing with the heart rate, creating a calming effect.

HOW TO PRACTICE

1. Inhale for five to six seconds.
2. Exhale for five to six seconds.
3. Keep the breath steady and rhythmic for 5–10 minutes.

Humming Bee Breath

This technique uses sound vibrations to soothe the nervous system and quiet the mind.

HOW TO PRACTICE

1. Inhale deeply through your nose.
2. Exhale while making a soft humming "mmm" sound.
3. Feel the vibration in your head and chest.
4. Repeat 5–10 times.

The 5-4-3-2-1 Technique

This technique enhances mindfulness through sensory awareness, helping to redirect your attention away from stressors and bring you back to the present moment. It encourages you to engage with your environment, calming your mind by focusing on sensory input.

HOW TO PRACTICE

1. Identify five things you can see around you.
2. Notice four things you can touch.
3. Acknowledge three sounds you can hear.
4. Recognize two scents you can smell.
5. Identify one thing you can taste.
6. Pair this with slow, controlled breaths, grounding you in the present.

The 5-4-3-2-1 technique is a simple mindfulness practice that grounds you in the present by engaging your senses. It effectively shifts focus from stress and anxiety, allowing for a calming reconnection with your surroundings.

Imagine you're in the middle of a high-pressure workday. You have back-to-back meetings, a looming deadline, and an inbox overflowing with emails. Feeling overwhelmed, you decide to take a moment to practice the 5-4-3-2-1 technique at your desk.

1. Identify five things you can see around you.

- ☐ The blue sticky notes on your monitor.
- ☐ The coffee mug that is half full.
- ☐ A potted plant sitting on the corner of your desk.
- ☐ Your coworker's colorful water bottle on the neighboring desk.
- ☐ The clock on the wall showing the time.

2. Notice four things you can touch.

- ☐ The smooth surface of your desk.
- ☐ The warmth of your coffee mug.
- ☐ The fabric of your chair.
- ☐ The keys of your keyboard.

3. Acknowledge three sounds you can hear.

- ☐ The quiet hum of the air-conditioning.
- ☐ The soft tapping of keyboards nearby.
- ☐ The muffled sound of voices from a distant meeting room.

4. Recognize two scents you can smell.

- ☐ The smell of coffee that has been freshly brewed.
- ☐ The hand sanitizer that you applied earlier in the day.

5. Identify one thing you can taste.

- ☐ Take a sip of your coffee and notice its taste.

6. Pair this with slow, controlled breaths, grounding you in the present.

As you move through each stop, you pair the exercise with slow, deep breaths, inhaling deeply through your nose and exhaling slowly through your mouth. By the end of the practice, you feel calmer and more focused, ready to tackle the next task on your to-do list.

Lion's Breath

This is a dynamic breathing technique that helps release tension and increase energy. It helps to make one's body feel energized and relieve tension in the jaw muscles.

HOW TO PRACTICE

1. Find a comfortable seated position, either resting on your heels or crossing your legs.
2. Place your palms firmly on your knees with your fingers spread apart.
3. Take a deep breath in through your nose and open your eyes as wide as possible.
4. Simultaneously, open your mouth fully and extend your tongue, directing the tip toward your chin.
5. Tighten the muscles at the front of your throat while exhaling through your mouth, producing a prolonged "haaa" sound.
6. Focus your gaze on the area between your eyebrows or the tip of your nose.
7. Repeat this breathing exercise two to three times.

Regular practice of Lion's Breath can enhance your energy and mental clarity. This dynamic technique boosts energy circulation while promoting relaxation, equipping you to tackle daily challenges with your newfound energy.

YOGA POSES FOR STRESS RELIEF

Integrating yoga into your daily routine is an effective method for alleviating stress, soothing your thoughts, and enhancing your overall health. These straightforward yoga poses are designed to engage both your body and mind, facilitating the release of tension and the attainment of equilibrium. Practicing these poses can significantly reduce your stress levels and promote relaxation.

Standing Forward Bend

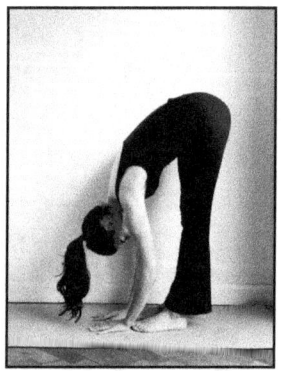

HOW TO PRACTICE

1. Stand tall with feet hip-width apart.
2. Exhale and slowly bend forward, keeping a slight bend in your knees.
3. Place your palms on the floor, letting your head rest against your legs.
4. Stretch your spine in different directions as you pull your head down.
5. For a deeper stretch, straighten your legs.
6. Hold for six to eight breaths.
7. Inhale, slowly raise your arms and torso back to standing.

The Standing Forward Bend promotes flexibility and relaxation. Following these steps helps release tension in your legs and back, allowing relaxation to envelop each part of your body.

Cat-Cow Pose

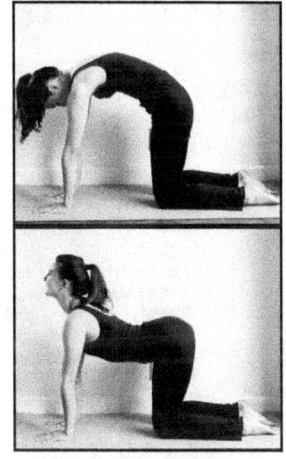

HOW TO PRACTICE

1. Start on all fours, with wrists directly under your shoulders and knees under your hips.
2. Inhale and hold your breath.
3. **Cat:** Exhale and round your back toward the ceiling, bringing your navel toward your spine.
4. Return to the neutral position with a straight back.
5. **Cow:** Inhale, tilt your pelvis back, and lift your tailbone up while drawing your navel in and keeping your spine aligned.
6. Continue to flow between Cat and Cow for several breaths.

Incorporating Cat-Cow Pose into your routine promotes spinal flexibility and relieves tension. This gentle flow enhances body awareness, making it an ideal exercise for relaxation and mindfulness.

Easy Pose

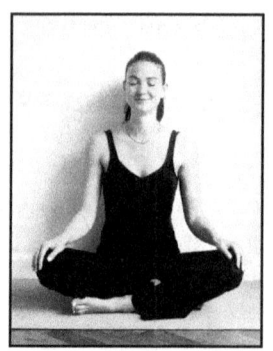

HOW TO PRACTICE

1. Sit on the floor with your legs extended in front of you.
2. Cross your legs, placing each foot beneath the opposite knee.
3. Rest your palms on your knees, with your fingers pointing down.
4. Align your head, neck, and spine, sitting upright with balanced weight.
5. Lengthen your spine while softening your neck, and gently relax your feet and thighs.
6. Stay for about a minute, then switch the cross of your legs.

Practicing Easy Pose fosters relaxation and mindfulness, enhancing your overall well-being. Regularly incorporating this pose into your routine can improve flexibility and aid in achieving mental clarity.

Bridge Pose

HOW TO PRACTICE

1. Lie on your back with knees bent and feet flat on the floor, hip-width apart.
2. Place your arms at your sides with palms facing down.
3. Inhale and lift your hips off the floor, rolling your spine up.
4. Squeeze your knees together to keep them aligned, and press your arms and shoulders into the floor to lift your chest.
5. Engage your legs and glutes to raise your hips higher.
6. Hold the pose for four to eight breaths, then slowly lower your hips back to the floor.

Bridge Pose is an excellent way to strengthen the back, glutes, and legs while promoting flexibility in the spine. Regular practice can enhance posture and relieve stress-related tension in the body.

Downward-Facing Dog

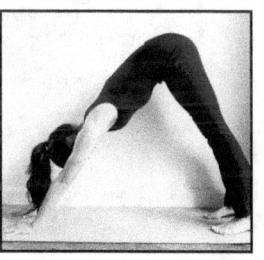

HOW TO PRACTICE

1. Start in a tabletop position.
2. Lift your hips up and back, forming an inverted V shape.
3. Keep your hands shoulder-width apart and press your heels toward the ground.
4. Hold for 5–10 breaths.

Reclining Butterfly

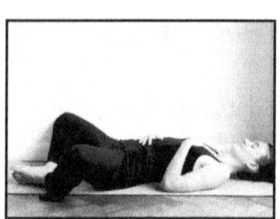

HOW TO PRACTICE

1. Lie on your back and bring the soles of your feet together.
2. Let your knees fall open like butterfly wings.
3. Place one hand on your heart and one on your belly, breathing deeply.

Supine Twist

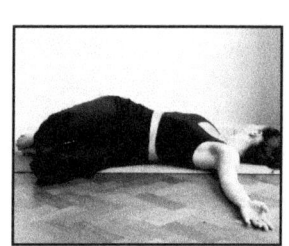

HOW TO PRACTICE

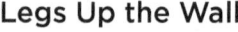

1. Lie on your back and bring one knee to your chest.
2. Gently twist the knee across your body while keeping your shoulders on the floor.
3. Extend your opposite arm and gaze in the opposite direction.
4. Hold for a few breaths, then switch sides.

Legs Up the Wall

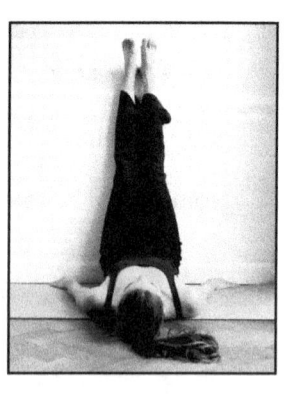

HOW TO PRACTICE

1. Sit sideways against a wall.
2. Swing your legs up and rest them against the wall.
3. Lie back with arms relaxed by your sides and breathe deeply.

Regular practice of these yoga poses leads to a reduction in stress and anxiety while enhancing both mental and physical health. Moving at your own pace and focusing on your breath is essential, as each pose helps to reconnect with your body and release any tension. With consistent practice, these simple yet effective poses become a vital part of your self-care routine, promoting peace and relaxation in your daily life.

COGNITIVE BEHAVIORAL THERAPY

Cognitive behavioral therapy (CBT) is a practical and highly effective approach to improving mental health. At its core, CBT is based on the idea that our thoughts, emotions, and behaviors are deeply interconnected. In simple terms, how we think shapes how we feel, and how we feel influences what we do. Negative or distorted thinking patterns can lead to emotional distress and unhelpful behaviors. CBT helps us identify these thought patterns, challenge them, and replace them with healthier, more realistic alternatives. This process can lead to improved emotional well-being, healthier behaviors, and greater resilience.

If you're new to the concept of self-help or CBT, don't worry! This section will break down the essential principles of CBT so you can start applying them to your own life. It will provide a clear understanding of how to recognize and assess your own thoughts and emotions, even if you don't have a background in psychology.

What Is CBT, and Why Is It Effective?

CBT is a therapeutic approach that focuses on the present, helping individuals identify and change negative thought patterns that contribute to emotional distress. By learning how to challenge and reframe these thoughts, individuals can change their emotional responses and behaviors. This method is evidence-based, meaning it has been proven to work for a variety of mental health conditions, including anxiety, depression, and stress.

Unlike some other therapeutic approaches, CBT is solution-focused and goal-oriented. It offers practical tools that can be applied in daily life, making it a great option for individuals seeking to make real changes in how they think, feel, and act.

How Can You Begin Using CBT?

The first step in using CBT is learning how to observe your thoughts. Most people aren't aware of the constant stream of thoughts that run through their minds, many of which can be negative or self-critical. CBT encourages you to pause and become aware of these thoughts, especially those that lead to negative emotions or behaviors.

This section will introduce you to a variety of CBT tools that you can begin using right away to help manage your thoughts, emotions, and behaviors. Each tool will be explained in simple terms, and you'll receive practical guidance on how to implement them into your daily life. Keep in mind that CBT is a skill, and like any skill, it improves with practice.

What to Expect in This Section

In this section, you'll get an introduction to some of the most effective CBT techniques. These techniques are designed to help you identify negative thought patterns, challenge them, and replace them with healthier alternatives. Visuals and simple examples will be provided to help reinforce each concept, and we'll also offer guidance on how to seek professional help if needed, especially if you find yourself struggling to implement these techniques on your own.

Whether you're starting your journey in mental health or simply want to gain more control over your emotional well-being, the tools in this section will give you the foundation you need to begin applying CBT in your life. By the end of this section, you'll have practical tools to help you improve emotional resilience and develop healthier thought patterns.

Unraveling Cognitive Distortions

One of the main goals of CBT is to identify and challenge cognitive distortions. These are irrational or biased ways of thinking that can negatively affect your emotions and behavior. By recognizing and unraveling these distortions, you can change your thinking patterns to be more balanced and rational.

HOW TO PRACTICE

1. Identify negative thoughts and assess if they fall into one of the common cognitive distortions:
   - ☐ **All-or-nothing thinking:** Viewing situations in black-and-white terms, with no middle ground
   - ☐ **Overgeneralization:** Drawing broad conclusions based on a single event or piece of evidence
   - ☐ **Catastrophizing:** Expecting the worst possible outcome in any situation
   - ☐ **Mental filtering:** Focusing on negative aspects while ignoring positive ones
2. Challenge the thought by asking if it is realistic or evidence-based.
3. Replace the distortion with a more balanced thought.

Example of This Technique

You feel left out because your friends are hanging out without you. You think, "They don't like me anymore, and I'll always be alone." This thought is an overgeneralization. You challenge it by remembering times when your friends have included you, and that one missed hangout doesn't define your entire friendship. You reframe the thought: "This is just one moment; I know my friends value me."

Cognitive Restructuring

Cognitive restructuring is the process of identifying and changing irrational or unhelpful thoughts. Once a negative thought or belief is recognized, it can be challenged and replaced with a more accurate, constructive perspective. This technique helps shift your mindset from self-criticism to self-compassion.

HOW TO PRACTICE

1. Identify a negative or irrational belief you hold about yourself or a situation.
2. Investigate the origins of this belief and whether it is based on evidence.
3. Challenge this belief by considering alternative, more realistic thoughts.
4. Replace the negative belief with a healthier one.

Example of This Technique

You have a big basketball game and think, "I'm terrible at sports. I'm going to embarrass myself." You challenge this thought by asking, "What proof do I have that I'm bad at sports? I've been practicing, and I've had good moments before." You replace the thought with: "I might not be perfect, but I can give my best effort and enjoy the game."

Exposure and Response Prevention

Exposure and response prevention (ERP) is a technique used to help teens confront and reduce anxiety, especially related to obsessive-compulsive behaviors. By slowly facing what you fear and resisting the urge to perform a comforting behavior, you can reduce anxiety over time.

HOW TO PRACTICE

1. Identify the situation that triggers your compulsive behavior (e.g., fear of germs).
2. Gradually expose yourself to the feared stimulus without engaging in the compulsive behavior (e.g., touching a doorknob but not washing your hands immediately).
3. Over time, your anxiety should lessen as you learn that the feared situation is not as harmful as it seems.

Example of This Technique

You're afraid of germs and feel the urge to wash your hands after touching things at school. Gradually, you expose yourself to this fear by touching things like the classroom desk or a doorknob and resisting the urge to wash your hands immediately. As you continue this, you realize that touching things doesn't make you sick, and the anxiety becomes more manageable.

Interoceptive Exposure

Interoceptive exposure is a technique that helps teens cope with anxiety related to physical sensations. Whether it's a racing heart, sweaty palms, or dizziness, learning to tolerate and accept these feelings can help you manage anxiety and panic attacks.

HOW TO PRACTICE

1. Identify the bodily sensations you fear (e.g., rapid heartbeat, dizziness).
2. Intentionally induce these sensations by engaging in activities like exercise.
3. Resist the urge to avoid or distract yourself from the sensations.
4. Practice mindfulness to observe the sensations without panic.

Example of This Technique

You're worried that exercising will make your heart race and lead to a panic attack. To challenge this fear, you jog for a few minutes, intentionally raising your heart rate. Instead of panicking, you observe your racing heart and remind yourself that this is temporary and harmless. Over time, you become more comfortable with these sensations.

Nightmare Exposure and Rescripting

Nightmares can be terrifying, but with a technique called rescripting, you can take control of your dreams. By changing the story of your nightmare, you can make it less frightening and empower yourself to feel safe during sleep.

HOW TO PRACTICE

1. Recall a recent nightmare and describe the emotion it evoked.
2. Work to alter the narrative of the nightmare, adding positive or empowering elements.
3. Visualize this new version of the nightmare before going to sleep.

Example of This Technique

You often have a nightmare where you're lost at school and can't find your friends. To rescript it, you imagine yourself calmly finding your friends, and everyone helps you figure out the way back. Before bed, you visualize this new ending, helping your mind associate calmness with the dream. Over time, the nightmare becomes less frequent and less scary.

Play the Script Until the End

This technique involves mentally facing your worst fears. By imagining your worst-case scenario and realizing that you can handle it, you can reduce the power it has over you. It's all about accepting uncertainty and being prepared for any outcome.

HOW TO PRACTICE

1. Identify the feared situation (e.g., public speaking).
2. Mentally imagine the worst-case scenario (e.g., forgetting your speech).
3. Visualize yourself handling the situation calmly and competently.
4. Recognize that even if the worst happens, you can cope with it.

Example of This Technique

You're nervous about giving a presentation in class and think, "What if I forget everything and make a fool of myself?" You play out the worst-case scenario where you forget your lines, but then you calmly recover by explaining your main points in a different way. You realize that even if you forget a few details, you can still present yourself confidently, and it won't be the end of the world.

CBT techniques serve as effective strategies for adolescents to cope with stress, anxiety, and disruptive thoughts. By consistently applying these methods, individuals can gain mastery over their emotional responses and cognitive processes, foster resilience, and tackle obstacles with enhanced self-assurance.

INCORPORATING MINDFULNESS IN DAILY LIFE

Mindfulness extends beyond meditation; it's a practice that can be integrated into our daily lives. It's about being present and aware of every activity. Whether you're brushing your teeth, preparing a meal, or walking to work, mindfulness can transform routines into moments of calm and clarity. We will explore practical ways to incorporate mindfulness into everyday tasks, reducing stress, enhancing focus, and appreciating life's simple moments. By making mindfulness a part of our daily activities, we can promote balance and well-being throughout the day.

Mindful Gardening

Gardening is an excellent way to practice mindfulness, allowing you to connect with nature while nurturing plants. As you dig your hands into the soil, sense the Earth's texture and temperature. Observe the vibrant colors of the flowers and the various shapes of the leaves. Each planting or weeding session can become a meditative practice where you focus on the rhythm of your movements and the process of nurturing life. The act of watering plants, feeling the weight of the watering can, and witnessing the growth over time helps create patience and appreciation for the natural world. For young adults seeking a therapeutic outlet, gardening can be a powerful way to ground themselves, reduce stress, and find joy in nurturing living things.

Mindful Eating

Mindful eating is a simple yet powerful way to change your relationship with food. This practice involves slowing down to truly appreciate the flavors, smells, and textures of what you consume. Picture this: Instead of mindlessly munching through meals or grabbing snacks on the go, you pause to savor every bite. Imagine biting into a crisp apple, feeling its texture, tasting its sweetness, and recognizing the energy and nourishment it provides. By focusing on these sensory experiences, you start to develop a deeper gratitude for food. This promotes healthier eating habits and helps reduce stress by grounding you in the present moment. In modern times, many of us eat while distracted by screens or in a hurry; mindful eating can serve as a gentle reminder to slow down and enjoy life's simpler pleasures (Mayo Clinic Staff, 2022).

Mindful Walking

Turning walking into a meditative exercise can significantly enhance your awareness of both movement and surroundings. Instead of walking solely as a means to get from point A to B, consider each step as an opportunity to engage with the world around you. Mindful walking isn't about covering long distances; it's about being fully present. As you walk, notice the sensation of your feet touching the ground, the rhythm of your breath syncing with your pace, and the feel of the air against your skin. This kind of walking allows you to reconnect with your body and environment, offering a respite from the constant buzz of thoughts and distractions. For young adults grappling with emotional challenges, adopting mindful walking can offer a much-needed break, promoting mental clarity and reducing stress (Wondermed, 2023).

Mindful Technology Use

In our digital age, where devices demand our constant attention, practicing mindful technology use becomes essential. This practice involves setting clear intentions before engaging with any device, whether it's your smartphone, tablet, or computer. Perhaps you're using them for entertainment, work, or staying connected. Whatever the purpose, be conscious of when and how long you plan to stay engaged. Establish boundaries, such as dedicating specific times for checking emails or social media, ensuring that your digital consumption doesn't overwhelm your real-life interactions. By doing so, you create boundaries that limit your digital activities, freeing up space for more intensive and mindful experiences that will increase your overall happiness and well-being. This approach is especially beneficial for teens and young adults who might otherwise find themselves endlessly scrolling through feeds, missing out on genuine human interactions or personal reflections. Encouraging mindful technology use is also a valuable strategy for parents aiming to support their children's development of emotional resilience and self-discipline (Mayo Clinic Staff, 2022).

STRESS-REDUCTION ACTIVITIES

Stress has become a common feature of modern life, often leaving us searching for effective ways to find relief. Fortunately, there are accessible and proven techniques to ease tension and promote calmness, each offering unique benefits for both the mind and body. Mindfulness practices, like coloring and nature connection, offer pathways to greater self-awareness, emotional balance, and inner peace.

Mindfulness coloring is an accessible outlet for stress reduction, particularly appealing due to its creative, nonverbal nature. Engaging in coloring demands attention to subtle details, whether it's selecting colors or creating intricate patterns. By focusing deeply on these activities, the mind becomes absorbed in the present moment, providing respite from external worries and anxieties. The process is inherently meditative, encouraging a state of flow where time seems to vanish and the mind finds a peaceful rhythm. Mindfulness coloring doesn't require any artistic skill, only a willingness to immerse oneself in a calming, creative endeavor.

Picture yourself returning home after a long, stressful day. You grab a detailed coloring book filled with floral designs, sit down with a set of colored pencils, and let yourself explore the simple joy of filling in each shape. As you choose vibrant colors and carefully shade each petal, your mind begins to quiet, and the stresses of the day fade into the background. This is the magic of adult coloring books—they offer you a creative escape and a way to center yourself. You don't need to be an artist; all that's required is your willingness to engage in the soothing process. As the patterns come to life under your hand, you'll find yourself feeling calmer, more focused, and maybe even a little accomplished.

Immersing oneself in nature offers a powerful means of emotional grounding and stress relief. Nature connection encourages individuals to spend time outdoors, observing the beauty and complexity of the natural environment. Whether walking through a forest, sitting by a river, or simply strolling in a local park, being outside allows one to engage fully with their surroundings. Pay attention to the sounds of birds, the rustle of leaves, and the fresh, earthy scents. Picture yourself stepping into a quiet forest trail, the sunlight filtering through the canopy above, casting a warm glow on the path ahead. You pause to listen to the melodic chirping of birds and take a deep breath, inhaling the fresh, earthy aroma of nature. In this moment, the weight of your responsibilities begins to lift, replaced by a soothing sense of presence.

Incorporating mindfulness into our lives helps manage stress, improve well-being, and encourage deeper connections. Mindful breathing, yoga, and daily practices build resilience and ease life's challenges. These techniques promote calmness, focus, and clarity, helping to maintain emotional balance during chaotic moments. With consistent practice, mindfulness becomes a natural routine, allowing us to face life with greater confidence.

As we transition into the next chapter, we will examine the essential skills that form the backbone of meaningful relationships and effective teamwork. Communication is more than exchanging words; it is about promoting understanding, trust, and collaboration. We will explore active listening techniques, the healthy expression of emotions, building empathy, and resolving conflicts—key elements that bridge gaps and strengthen bonds.

KEY TAKEAWAYS

- **Emotional burdens:** Acknowledge the emotional weights we carry, such as guilt and anxiety, to begin the healing process and foster personal growth.

- **Resilience:** Build emotional resilience to better handle life's challenges. This involves understanding societal pressures, adopting a growth mindset, and cultivating supportive relationships.

- **Self-awareness:** Enhance personal growth and authenticity by cultivating self-awareness through techniques like mind mapping, values clarification, and seeking feedback.

- **Self-acceptance:** Embrace self-acceptance by challenging societal standards of beauty and success, and instead, focus on your own definitions while celebrating your individuality.

- **Mindful techniques:** Integrate mindfulness practices like deep breathing, yoga, and mindfulness in everyday activities to reduce stress and improve emotional well-being.

- **Cognitive behavioral techniques:** Use CBT methods to identify and reframe negative thought patterns, promoting emotional regulation and resilience.

- **Healthy relationships:** Foster and maintain positive, supportive friendships that encourage growth and enhance emotional well-being. Be mindful of toxic relationships and distance yourself from them.

- **Setting boundaries:** Establish and communicate clear personal boundaries to safeguard your emotional health and ensure mutual respect in relationships.

- **Stress management:** Engage in stress-reduction activities, such as mindfulness coloring or spending time in nature, to promote emotional balance and inner peace.

CHAPTER 8

Communication and Connection

Effective communication is the foundation
of every meaningful connection.

At the foundation of every meaningful connection, whether with family, friends, or colleagues, lies effective communication. Engaging in sincere dialogue allows us to connect on deeper levels, fostering empathy and trust that enrich our interactions and establish authentic bonds. By prioritizing the quality of our communication, we can transform our relationships into pillars of support, happiness, and personal growth, enriching our lives and nurturing a sense of inner peace.

ACTIVE LISTENING TECHNIQUES

Building strong relationships starts with understanding and validating each other's perspectives. Active listening is a powerful way to do this. When someone truly feels heard, it creates a sense of trust and safety in the relationship. Giving your full attention to what the other person is saying shows that you care, and this respect helps deepen the connection. It's not just about hearing words—it's about engaging with the emotions and thoughts behind them. When people feel understood, they're more likely to open up in return, creating a positive cycle of communication and mutual respect that strengthens the bond over time.

Active listening involves various techniques that go beyond merely hearing words. Employing strategies like paraphrasing, nodding, and asking open-ended questions not only demonstrates empathy but also keeps the conversation dynamic and meaningful (Cuncic, 2024). For instance, when you paraphrase a friend's concerns, you validate their feelings, showing that you value and understand their perspective. An affirmative nod or an inquisitive follow-up question, such as "Can you tell me more about that?" signals genuine interest, encouraging the other person to express themselves freely and fully.

However, effective active listening requires overcoming certain barriers. Distractions, biases, and emotions can cloud one's ability to remain fully present during conversations. Recognizing these obstacles is the first step toward maintaining focus. For example, busy environments or internal distractions, such as thinking ahead about how to respond, can interrupt the flow of attentive listening. Acknowledging personal biases that might influence how we interpret someone else's message is essential to keep our focus purely on understanding their viewpoint.

Emotions play a significant role in communication. If one is preoccupied with personal emotional turmoil, it can be challenging to listen actively. Being aware of one's emotional state and setting it aside can help keep attention on the speaker's words. Techniques such as mindful breathing or taking a moment to mentally prepare before engaging in a conversation can significantly improve attentiveness.

To truly master active listening, practice is key. Role-playing scenarios can provide valuable opportunities to hone this skill. Engaging in mock conversations with peers or participating in workshops where feedback is provided helps refine one's listening abilities. Such exercises allow individuals to explore different conversational dynamics and receive constructive feedback on their listening habits (Taylor, 2023).

Feedback from others serves as a mirror reflecting areas of improvement. It can highlight tendencies such as interrupting or failing to ask clarifying questions. With this insight, one can consciously work on enhancing these aspects, leading to more meaningful interactions.

The practice of active listening goes hand in hand with another critical component—validation. Validation involves acknowledging the other person's feelings and experiences without necessarily agreeing with them. This bridges emotional gaps and reinforces the speaker's feeling of being respected and valued. Simple affirmations like "I understand why you feel that way" can greatly enhance the relational bond by showing empathy and acceptance.

A great exercise to try is having group discussions where everyone takes turns practicing reflective listening. In these conversations, the listener simply repeats back what they've heard, summarizing the key points to make sure they understood correctly. This small act of reflection helps the speaker feel truly heard and understood. Over time, these practices can make a big difference in building stronger, more genuine connections with others.

Additionally, creating safe spaces for open expression promotes honest and effective communication. Creating an environment where individuals feel comfortable sharing their thoughts and emotions without fear of judgment or dismissal can lead to deeper, more connected relationships. Establishing ground rules for respectful dialogue in group settings can further support active listening practices.

Building strong relationships relies on active listening and validation. By giving full attention, using techniques like paraphrasing, and overcoming distractions, we deepen connections based on trust and empathy. Practicing these skills through feedback strengthens communication and promotes mutual respect, leading to more authentic relationships.

EXPRESSING EMOTIONS HEALTHILY

Honest expression of feelings is a huge part of building meaningful relationships, and it begins with identifying and naming our emotions. Understanding what we are feeling enables us to articulate those feelings better, aiding in self-regulation and enhancing communication during discussions. When we can name our emotions, it becomes easier to convey thoughts clearly, reducing misunderstandings that often arise from unclear or misinterpreted emotional signals. Emotional awareness extends beyond individual growth; it enhances interpersonal connections, making conversations more respectful and understanding.

Using "I" statements is a powerful technique for open and nondefensive communication. For instance, saying, "I feel upset when plans change at the last minute" focuses on the speaker's feelings rather than blaming the other person, which could lead to defensiveness. This approach promotes vulnerability and honesty, facilitating deeper connections. Vulnerability allows individuals to share their true selves, ensuring an environment where both parties feel safe to express themselves without fear of judgment. Schmitz (2016) highlights the importance of empathy and understanding in communication, as they provide valuable insights into others' emotions and contribute to building trust in relationships.

The impact of suppressed emotions can be detrimental, leading to the buildup of resentment and potential conflict. Holding back feelings might seem like an easier path initially, but it often results in tension and unresolved issues. Instead, expressing emotions helps release these feelings and contributes positively to mental well-being. Acknowledging and openly sharing emotions helps prevent minor disagreements from escalating into bigger conflicts.

Engaging in artistic activities can channel one's emotions creatively, allowing individuals to process their feelings in a meaningful way. One such creative activity is origami, the Japanese art of paper folding. For example, a person feeling stressed or anxious could fold a paper crane, which is traditionally seen as a symbol of peace and hope. As they carefully follow each step, the repetitive motion of folding the paper helps calm the mind and turn chaotic thoughts into something structured and beautiful. Through the process of transforming a simple piece of paper into a meaningful shape, individuals can channel their emotions and find emotional relief in creativity.

Additionally, therapy or counseling provides a structured environment for exploring emotions. Professionals guide individuals through the process of recognizing and articulating feelings, offering support and techniques for managing emotional expression effectively. In group discussions, participants can learn from each other's experiences, gaining new perspectives on expressing emotions within a supportive community. These activities promote self-awareness, an important component of emotional intelligence, which is vital for personal growth and building connections with others.

Developing these skills requires practice and a willingness to confront your emotions honestly. Embracing emotion-oriented conversations builds resilience, helping individuals manage complex emotional landscapes with ease. Emotional awareness and expression are journeys of self-discovery that are integral to maintaining authenticity in relationships.

RESOLVING CONFLICTS

Effective communication is not just about exchanging words; it serves as a robust mechanism for promoting relationships and addressing disputes. When individuals approach disagreements with a constructive mindset, they can turn potential conflicts into opportunities to build deeper connections and gain a better understanding of each other. The key is to identify the underlying causes of the disagreement, which leads to effective resolutions and helps minimize the likelihood of similar issues arising in the future.

Conflicts often arise from misunderstandings, unfulfilled needs, or differing values. Recognizing the fundamental causes necessitates a willingness to investigate deeper issues instead of merely concentrating on superficial disagreements. Acknowledging these essential concerns enables individuals to develop solutions that tackle the core of the conflict, resulting in more satisfying outcomes for everyone involved (*5 Conflict Resolution Strategies,* 2024).

For example, two friends might argue about where to go for dinner, but the real issue could be one friend's desire to feel heard and valued in the decision-making process. On the surface, it seems like a simple disagreement about food preferences, but the friend may feel overlooked or dismissed in past decisions. They may want to consider their input not just in choosing dinner but in other aspects of the relationship as well.

The other friend might not realize this underlying concern and could be taking the lead out of habit or convenience. If both friends take the time to communicate openly, they can uncover this deeper issue. The solution might involve taking turns choosing restaurants or checking in with each other before making decisions, ensuring both feel heard.

Once the root cause is identified, bargaining techniques become essential tools in conflict resolution. This process is not about "winning" but finding common ground that respects everyone's perspectives. Effective negotiation involves listening actively, clearly expressing needs, and seeking win-win solutions where possible. A sincere apology, when appropriate, is vital for restoring trust. Apologizing sincerely—without making excuses—demonstrates humility and a commitment to the relationship. It shows an understanding of how your actions may have impacted the other person and a willingness to make amends (Shonk, 2025).

Empathy is also important in managing conflicts. When each person understands the other's perspective, they gain insights into the emotions behind differing viewpoints. Empathy goes beyond mere sympathy; it involves deeply experiencing what another person feels, which lessens hostility and encourages genuine conversation. For instance, if a parent understands their child's frustration about curfew rules, they are more likely to reach a compromise that balances safety and freedom, addressing the concerns of both parties.

Incorporating empathy into conflict resolution practices changes the dynamic from adversarial to collaborative. People are more inclined to lower their defenses and work toward mutually beneficial solutions when they feel understood. Empathy doesn't always come naturally, especially in heated situations. Thus, it often requires conscious effort and practice, akin to exercising a muscle to strengthen it over time.

Additionally, regular reflection after real conflict experiences can provide valuable learning opportunities. Consider maintaining a journal to document disagreements and the steps taken to resolve them. Reflecting on past challenges helps clarify what worked and what didn't, promoting ongoing personal growth in handling disagreements.

For educators and wellness practitioners, guiding youth through such practical exercises empowers them to handle conflicts with greater confidence and competence. When adults create safe spaces for young people to explore and practice these skills, they help equip them with the resilience necessary for building stronger relationships throughout their lives.

Effective conflict resolution is a continuous journey of learning and growth. As we face new challenges and evolve as individuals, our approach to disagreements naturally changes. Staying open to feedback and being willing to adjust our strategies allows us to develop these essential skills further. This ongoing process helps create environments where communication thrives, encouraging stronger and more harmonious relationships in all areas of life.

BUILDING EMPATHY

In the previous section, we talked about the importance of empathy, and one way to nurture those skills is through reading, volunteer work, and discussions. Books and stories open a window into diverse lives, challenges, and emotions, offering a unique chance to walk in another person's shoes without leaving the comfort of your home. Through reading, you are not just learning about characters and plots; you're acquiring insights into human emotions and responses, which enhances your capacity for empathy. Similarly, volunteering exposes you to different life experiences and personal challenges, cultivating a shared sense of humanity. Discussing these experiences, whether over dinner or in study groups, further broadens empathetic understanding and creates shared experiences, uniting people from different walks of life in mutual growth.

Despite its importance, several barriers can make it difficult to empathize with others. Awareness of stereotypes, burnout, and cultural differences is important in overcoming these obstacles. Stereotypes, often unconsciously adopted, cloud judgment and create biases that prevent genuine connection. Recognizing and challenging these patterns is important. Alongside this, burnout can diminish empathy, especially when individuals are emotionally drained or overwhelmed. Taking time to tune into personal needs and practicing self-care can preserve one's empathic abilities. Additionally, embracing cultural differences instead of seeing them as impediments can enhance empathy. Recognizing and valuing diversity enables us to embrace a variety of perspectives, cultivating deeper understanding and acceptance.

Practical strategies can also reinforce ongoing empathetic connections. Using supportive language during conversations shows consideration and compassion, encouraging others to share openly. Simple phrases like "I understand how you feel" or "That sounds really tough" can affirm a person's feelings and promote a sense of safety and validation. Regular check-ins with friends, family, or colleagues are another way to maintain strong, empathetic ties. These don't have to be elaborate or time-consuming; even a quick message asking "How are you doing?" can make someone feel valued and heard. Consistent efforts to communicate empathetically contribute significantly to stronger, more resilient connections.

Empathy is important for both personal and community spheres. In communities, empathy ensures an environment where inclusivity and trust thrive, enabling individuals to work together toward common goals. Empathetic interactions within communities encourage openness, reduce conflicts, and inspire collective progress. Just as in personal relationships, where empathy promotes emotional well-being by creating bonds of understanding and love, in larger settings, it acts as a catalyst for innovation and positive change.

Empathy is a powerful tool for personal growth and emotional challenges. Developing empathy helps individuals gain a deeper understanding of their own emotions as well as those of others, which encourages stronger relationships and improves emotional resilience. Encouraging youth to participate in empathy-building activities, such as team sports or group projects, can help them practice putting themselves in others' shoes. These experiences not only develop their social skills but also teach teamwork and cooperation, reinforcing the importance of empathy in everyday interactions.

Parents and guardians also make a significant contribution toward empathetic values. By demonstrating empathetic behavior and promoting settings that encourage open expression and active listening, parents can help instill these skills in their children. Witnessing their parents address conflicts with empathy teaches children important lessons about managing their emotions and empathizing with others. Discussing feelings, acknowledging emotions, and practicing gratitude at home establishes a strong foundation for empathy to develop.

Educators and wellness practitioners are important in extending these teachings beyond the home environment. By integrating empathy training into their educational programs or counseling sessions, they equip young individuals with the necessary tools for developing emotional intelligence and strong relationships. Workshops and seminars centered on perspective-taking and compassion can motivate students to face life's challenges with empathy, turning difficulties into chances for growth and connection.

An Example of Building Empathy in Schools

Mrs. Thompson, a middle school teacher, knew that empathy was a critical life skill her students needed to develop. Hoping it would encourage understanding, connection, and emotional growth, she introduced a "Story Sharing" activity into her classroom.

THE STORY OF ANNA

One day, Anna, a quiet and reserved student, volunteered to share her story. Anna had been at the school for just a few months and had struggled with making friends. She explained how, during her first week, she tried to join a group during lunch but felt ignored. She mentioned how she overheard a few students whispering about her clothes and accent, which made her feel like an outsider.

"I just wanted to fit in," Anna said softly, her eyes glancing down at her hands. "But it felt like no one even noticed me."

Mrs. Thompson, creating a safe and supportive environment, asked the class, "How do you think Anna might have felt in that moment?"

A few students raised their hands to share their thoughts. "It must have been lonely," said Ethan. "I can't imagine how hard it would be to be new and feel like no one wants to talk to you."

"I'd feel really sad," added Mia, a classmate who had recently experienced her own struggles fitting in after moving to the area.

As the class listened attentively and empathized with Anna's experience, something shifted in the room. The students were no longer just classmates—they were peers who understood one another's vulnerabilities.

After Anna finished her story, Mrs. Thompson facilitated a discussion on how to make the classroom more inclusive. She asked, "What can we do to make sure someone like Anna feels seen and heard?"

Slowly, ideas began to flow:

- "We could ask new students to join us during lunch," suggested Liam.
- "Maybe we could make an effort to include people when we're working on group projects," Mia added.
- "I'll make sure to speak up if I see someone sitting alone," said Ethan.

Anna's story opened the door to not only understanding her feelings but also tangible actions that could improve the classroom dynamic. By the end of the session, Mrs. Thompson could see a subtle yet important shift. The students became more mindful of each other, and a newfound sense of community began to emerge.

Through the simple act of sharing personal stories, Anna's experience helped her classmates better understand the impact of exclusion and the importance of kindness. Story sharing had fostered empathy, turning a moment of vulnerability into a collective opportunity for growth and compassion. Mrs. Thompson knew that creating space for these types of conversations would lead to lasting positive change, making the classroom a place where every student felt valued and heard.

Effective communication is essential for encouraging strong relationships in all aspects of life. Focusing on active listening, expressing emotions healthily, resolving conflicts, and showing empathy enables individuals to improve their interactions and forge deeper connections with others. These skills lead to better understanding and collaboration while contributing to personal growth and emotional intelligence. Building meaningful relationships paves the way for support, joy, and collective progress, enriching our lives in countless ways. Ultimately, the journey of improving communication and connection is a continuous process, enabling us to thrive both personally and within our communities.

EMPATHY JOURNALING ACTIVITY

Take your time to reflect on each empathy journaling prompt. Find a quiet moment to think without distractions. Read the prompt carefully and let your thoughts flow freely. Write your responses candidly, expressing your feelings and insights honestly. Focus on your personal experiences, as there are no right or wrong answers. You may jot down related emotions or memories that come to mind. After responding, review your thoughts to see how they can enhance your understanding and practice of empathy in daily life.

Think about a book or show that helped you understand someone else's life better. What did you learn about the character's feelings or struggles? How did it change the way you think about understanding others in real life?

_____

_____

_____

_____

_____

_____

_____

_____

_____

_____

_____

_____

Remember a recent time when you met or talked to people from a different background. What did you learn from them?
How did it help you understand their life and make you more empathetic?

_____

_____

_____

_____

_____

_____

_____

_____

_____

_____

_____

_____

Think of a time when it was hard to understand someone because of a stereotype or assumption. What did you do to see things differently? What did you learn about yourself, and how can that help you be more understanding in the future?

_____

_____

_____

_____

_____

_____

_____

_____

_____

_____

_____

_____

KEY TAKEAWAYS

- Building meaningful connections relies on effective communication, which nurtures empathy, trust, and personal growth in relationships.

- Techniques such as paraphrasing, nodding, and asking open-ended questions can improve understanding and validation, strengthening emotional bonds.

- It's important to overcome distractions, biases, and personal emotions to stay focused and attentive during conversations.

- Acknowledging and validating others' feelings helps build stronger relationships by showing empathy and acceptance.

- Being honest about your feelings is vital for building relationships. Using "I" statements encourages vulnerability and reduces defensiveness.

- Understanding the underlying causes of conflicts and communicating effectively can help resolve disagreements constructively, deepening connections.

- Cultivating empathy through activities like reading, volunteering, and open discussions improves understanding and strengthens relationships.

- Recognizing the traits of healthy friendships—such as mutual respect, support, and understanding—contributes to personal growth and emotional well-being.

- Identifying and addressing toxic behaviors in relationships is essential for mental health, and setting boundaries can protect against negative influences.

- Journaling to explore empathy can promote reflection and personal growth, helping individuals practice empathy in their daily interactions.

- Developing communication and empathy is an ongoing process that enriches both personal relationships and the community, fostering emotional intelligence and shared growth.

Conclusion

Emotions play an important role in shaping our experiences, especially during the journey of growing up. For teens and young adults, navigating personal growth while managing a range of complex emotions can be particularly challenging. This book is designed to offer support, providing tools to understand and manage emotional burdens effectively. It's designed not only for those facing these struggles but also for parents, guardians, educators, and wellness practitioners who want to guide and support young people in building emotional resilience and intelligence.

Recognizing and understanding the weight of emotional burdens is a critical first step. These feelings often show up in unexpected ways, influencing how we view ourselves and interact with others. Acknowledging them allows us to see that emotions are not fleeting but powerful forces that shape our reality. Once we become aware of these emotions, we begin the path to healing and growth. Even small steps forward can lead to meaningful changes, turning what once seemed overwhelming into manageable parts.

Emotional resilience is the key to managing life's fluctuations. It encompasses our ability to recover from failures, adapt to challenges, and advance with renewed vigor. Fostering emotional resilience transforms obstacles into avenues for personal development, whether confronting academic demands, social challenges, or individual hardships. By establishing effective strategies and coping techniques, we can approach difficulties with assurance, recognizing that resilience empowers us to endure any trial.

Mindfulness is another key element in the pursuit of emotional well-being. By incorporating mindfulness practices like breathing exercises and meditation into our daily lives, we can reduce stress and gain clarity. These practices encourage us to stay present, letting go of judgment and external pressures. As we embrace mindfulness, we can experience a deeper sense of calm and a stronger and more meaningful connection with ourselves and the world around us.

Self-acceptance complements mindfulness by nurturing a positive self-image. In a world often driven by comparison, embracing who we are and accepting our unique qualities brings relief from self-doubt. Understanding that we each have our own path helps us appreciate our individuality rather than seeing our differences as shortcomings. Practicing self-compassion encourages inner peace and genuine confidence, allowing us to silence negative self-talk and celebrate our strengths.

This book is filled with insights, exercises, and strategies designed to help teens, parents, educators, and wellness practitioners develop emotional resilience, practice mindfulness, and embrace self-acceptance. These interconnected elements serve to strengthen emotional intelligence and overall well-being, making it easier to navigate life's challenges with a sense of purpose and clarity.

The journey ahead is one of ongoing growth. Embracing these principles doesn't mean that challenges will disappear, but it does provide the tools to handle them in a healthy, constructive way. The ultimate goal is to become stronger, more self-aware, and capable of living a life aligned with your values and aspirations. Let's take this journey together—unlocking the potential within to thrive and flourish in an ever-evolving world.

Financial Literacy for Independence

Understanding financial principles is a fundamental step to gaining peace of mind and confidence in managing your money.

Enhancing our financial understanding is important for achieving inner peace. Enter into the realm of finances, where each decision can either encourage tranquility or induce anxiety. Picture yourself empowered and self-assured while discussing finances and adept at handling unforeseen expenses. This chapter presents fundamental aspects of financial literacy, equipping us with the essential tools to maneuver through the intricacies of wealth management with ease. By learning about concepts such as revenue, holdings, and debts, we can redefine our connection with money and move toward a more stable and fulfilling future.

UNDERSTANDING FINANCIAL BASICS

Grasping fundamental financial concepts is essential for young adults who want to manage their money effectively. At the heart of financial literacy is an understanding of key terms, including income, expenses, assets, and liabilities. These concepts serve as the foundation for making informed financial decisions. For example, knowing how to track your income is a powerful tool. Income isn't limited to just your paycheck; it includes various types, such as earned, passive, and portfolio income. *Earned income* is the money you earn through your job or services you provide, while *passive income* is money you earn without actively working on what is generating the income. A person may put in some effort upfront, but after the initial effort, that income comes in regularly with minimal effort in maintaining the project that generates it. *Portfolio income* includes earnings from dividends and interest earned on different types of accounts, such as savings accounts or capital gains from your investments. Understanding these different income streams helps you create a more comprehensive budget, enabling you to not only manage your finances but also set yourself up for long-term financial success.

Understanding expenses means knowing where and how your money exits your wallet. Expenses can be categorized broadly into fixed, variable, and discretionary types, helping you prioritize spending. Fixed expenses are those that do not change every month, such as rent or mortgage payments; they remain consistent for long periods of time. Variable expenses are expenses that change from month to month; for example, grocery amounts change each month. Discretionary expenses are the nonessential items one chooses to buy, such as a Netflix subscription.

Assets and liabilities are important concepts to understand when it comes to managing your money. Assets are things you own that have value. This could include things like your car, the money in your savings account, or investments like stocks or bonds. Assets help build your wealth and can increase your financial security. Some assets, such as a house or rental property, can also bring in extra money over time.

Liabilities are what you owe, like loans, credit card debt, or a mortgage.

They are amounts you'll need to pay back later. Liabilities take money away from you, which lowers your wealth. It's important to manage debt effectively because having too much can become difficult to handle. The goal is to grow your assets while reducing what you owe whenever you can.

Financial literacy encourages confidence in financial discussions, greatly alleviating money-related anxieties. While open conversations about finances may initially seem intimidating, a solid understanding of financial concepts allows individuals to engage more comfortably and assertively. Topics such as budgeting, investing, and saving can be approached with peers or advisors with increased ease and productivity. These topics will be expanded upon further in the next section.

BUDGETING AND SAVING STRATEGIES

Understanding how to manage money is one of the most important skills you can learn as a teenager. You might not realize it now, but the decisions you make with your money today will affect your financial future. Whether you're saving for a new phone, a trip, or just learning to manage your income, budgeting is the key to making the most of your money. Here's a breakdown of how you can approach budgeting, along with some examples that are relatable to your life right now.

- **Wants:** These are nonessential items or services that enhance your quality of life but are not necessary for survival. Examples include luxury items, entertainment, and dining out.

- **Needs:** These are essential requirements for basic survival and well-being. Needs usually include food, shelter, clothing, healthcare, and education.

- **Investments:** Investments refer to assets purchased with the expectation of earning a return or appreciation over time. This can include stocks, real estate, bonds, and mutual funds. Investments help grow wealth and secure financial stability for the future.

- **Savings:** Savings involve setting aside money for future use, typically in a safe and easily accessible account. This can include emergency funds, retirement funds, or money for specific goals such as travel or education. Savings are important for financial security and can help cover unexpected expenses.

Needs

HOUSING (25%-35%)

Housing expenses are typically associated with rent or living costs. For teenagers, you might not be paying rent yet, but if you contribute to family bills or your living situation requires you to pitch in, it's important to start thinking about this.

EXAMPLE

If you're helping your parents with household bills, or if you pay for your own room, aim to spend 25%-35% of your income. For example:

- If you earn $500 a month, you could contribute $125-$175 toward household expenses.

INSURANCE (10%-20%)

Insurance helps protect you against unexpected costs like health care or car expenses. As a teenager, you may not yet pay for health or car insurance, but you may contribute to your family's policy, or you might need insurance for your own car if you're driving.

EXAMPLE

Let's say you're working a part-time job and earning $500 a month. You should consider setting aside 10%-20% of that for insurance.

- $50 to $100 could go toward contributing to car insurance or your health insurance.

FOOD (10%–15%)

Food costs include groceries, snacks, and dining out. As a teenager, this is an area where it's easy to overspend if you eat out frequently. But with some planning, you can enjoy eating while staying within your budget.

EXAMPLE

If you allocate 10%–15% of your income to food, it could look something like this:

- If you earn $500 a month, you'd have $50–$75 for groceries or takeout.
- You could plan your meals for the week, cook at home, and save money for those weekends when you might want to grab a bite with friends.

TRANSPORT (10%–15%)

Transportation costs refer to any expenses related to getting around, like gas, bus fares, or public transit passes. If you don't drive yet, your transportation options might just include a bus or metro card, but it's still important to budget for it.

EXAMPLE

Allocate 10%–15% of your income for transportation.

- If you earn $500 a month, set aside $50–$75 for transport.
- If you rely on public transportation, a monthly pass could fall within that range. If you have a car, that money could be used for gas or maintenance.

MEDICAL (5%–10%)

Medical expenses include things like doctor visits, over-the-counter medications, and even gym memberships. Staying healthy is important, and having a budget for these expenses ensures you're covered when you need them.

EXAMPLE

Set aside 5%–10% for medical expenses.

- If you earn $500, that's $25–$50 to cover any health-related costs.

SAVINGS (10%–15%)

Saving money is important for your future. Setting aside a portion of your income for savings means you're building a financial cushion that can help in case of emergencies or fund future goals like college or a car.

EXAMPLE

Try to save 10%–15% of your income. For instance:

- If you earn $500 a month, try saving $50–$75.
- This could be used to build an emergency fund or for a specific goal, like a new phone or a future trip with friends.

Wants

PERSONAL (5%–10%)

Personal expenses cover anything that helps you feel good or take care of yourself, such as clothes, personal care items, or entertainment.

EXAMPLE

Budget 5%–10% of your income for personal expenses.

- If you earn $500 a month, you can spend $25–$50 on things like new clothes or a haircut.

RECREATION (5%-10%)

Recreation includes fun activities like going to the movies, hanging out with friends, or attending events. Budgeting for fun ensures you can enjoy life without feeling guilty about spending money.

EXAMPLE

Set aside 5%–10% for recreation.

- $25–$50 of your $500 income could go toward activities like movies, concerts, or weekend trips.

GIVING (10%-15%)

Giving back to your community or supporting causes you care about is an important part of financial responsibility. It doesn't have to be a huge amount, but setting aside a little money to donate or help out is a great habit to form.

EXAMPLE

If you allocate 10%–15% for giving, that's $50–$75 out of your $500 income.

- You could donate this to a local charity or even use it to help a friend in need.

CLOTHING (2%-5%)

Clothing expenses include the purchase of new clothes, shoes, or accessories. New clothes can be considered a want or a need depending on the intention behind the purchase. If you need clothes because yours no longer fit, or if they are not appropriate for specific events, then that's a reason to purchase new clothes, and it would be considered a need. If you purchase new clothes because you want a new brand, such as Nike, that would be considered a want. This is one area where you can keep costs down by shopping smart and taking advantage of sales or discounts.

EXAMPLE
Budget 2%-5% for clothing.

- If you earn $500, that's $10-$25 for new clothes or shoes.

By budgeting early, you'll develop strong financial habits that will set you up for a stable and successful future. Budgeting isn't just about restricting your spending—it's about making smart, intentional choices with your money so you can enjoy life now while preparing for the future!

Tips For Saving Money

Saving money during your teenage years can be straightforward. It involves making informed spending choices while still enjoying your youth. Whether you choose cash for smaller transactions or utilize student discounts, these strategies will enhance your financial management skills and help you save for future goals. Let's examine some practical methods to begin!

- **Use cash for essential purchases**
  Paying with cash for necessary items can help you manage your expenditures because physically handing over money feels more significant than using a card.

  EXAMPLE Withdraw a fixed amount of cash at the week's start for essentials like food, transport, or minor shopping. Once that cash is spent, additional purchases aren't possible.

- **Review your budget consistently**
  Regular budget checks help keep you accountable, allowing adjustments for any income or expense changes while highlighting areas for potential savings.

  EXAMPLE At the end of each week or month, assess your expenditures to determine if you adhered to your budget or overshot in certain categories. Revise your budget for the upcoming month based on your findings.

- **Cancel unused subscriptions**
  Unused subscriptions can quietly deplete your finances. Eliminating those you don't use frees up resources for essential expenses or savings.

  EXAMPLE If you're not actively using a subscription service, terminate it. The additional $10–15 monthly can either bolster your savings or fund a more significant need.

- **Establish a "fun fund" for leisure spending**
  Creating a designated fund enables you to save specifically for enjoyable or nonessential purchases while maintaining your budget.

  EXAMPLE Allocate $20 per month to your "fun fund" for leisure activities such as concerts, film outings, or shopping. Once you reach your savings goal, indulge without guilt or financial strain.

- **Uncover free sources of enjoyment**
  Engaging in free activities allows you to have fun without straining your finances.

  EXAMPLE Instead of shelling out money on entertainment, seek free community events, local parks, or nearby libraries. Alternatively, host a game night or potluck dinner with friends rather than dining out.

- **Limit impulse shopping**
  Impulsive shopping sprees can derail your budget, especially when motivated by boredom or stress. Setting boundaries helps you stay financially grounded.

EXAMPLE Prior to shopping, create a detailed list of items you genuinely need and establish a spending cap. If the impulse to splurge arises, take a moment to reconsider whether those items are truly necessary, maintaining adherence to your budget.

- **Save bonuses and unexpected income**
  The extra money from gifts, bonuses, or allowances presents an excellent opportunity to save without hindering your regular budget.

  EXAMPLE If you receive a $50 gift, think about saving $40 and allocating $10 for a small treat to enjoy.

- **Implement a cash envelope system**
  The cash envelope strategy involves designating specific cash amounts into labeled envelopes for various categories like food, entertainment, and transportation.

  EXAMPLE Start the week with $100 and allocate it into three envelopes: $50 for groceries, $30 for transport, and $20 for entertainment. Once an envelope is depleted, additional spending in that category waits until the following week.

- **Cook meals instead of dining out**
  Preparing your meals can be significantly more cost-effective than eating at restaurants or ordering takeout.

  EXAMPLE Rather than spending $10 each day on fast food, making lunch at home might only cost $3–$4. This can lead to savings of over $30 a week, which you can contribute to your savings or use for other needs.

- **Set financial goals for various time frames**
  Establishing both short-term and long-term financial goals provides direction and helps mitigate overspending.

  > **EXAMPLE**
  > **Short-term goal:** Save $100 for an enjoyable outing with friends within the next month.
  > **Long-term goal:** Accumulate $500 within six months to purchase a new phone.

- **Regularly monitor your bank balance**
  Keeping track of your bank account prevents unexpected surprises and overdrafts.

  > **EXAMPLE** Utilize a banking app to check your account balance every few days. If your funds are running low, consider delaying nonessential purchases until you have more money available.

- **Resist peer pressure to spend**
  Social influence can encourage unnecessary spending, but staying committed to your budget and financial aspirations helps you steer clear of these traps.

  > **EXAMPLE** If friends propose attending a costly concert that you can't afford, explain your situation politely and suggest exploring lower-cost or free options together.

- **Capitalize on student discounts**
  Many retailers and online platforms provide discounts to students. Utilizing these can significantly reduce your expenses on essential and desired items.

EXAMPLE Present your student ID at stores and restaurants to access discounts. Various streaming services and tech companies often offer special student pricing that can reduce your monthly financial burdens.

Embracing these approaches can greatly improve your financial health. By being aware of your spending patterns and making informed choices, you can effectively save money while enjoying life. Whether through a dedicated fun fund or taking advantage of discounts, small adjustments lead to substantial financial growth.

FINANCIAL GOAL SETTING

Setting and achieving financial goals play a vital role in attaining financial independence. These goals serve as a road map, guiding individuals toward a secure and prosperous financial future. Learning to identify, plan, and monitor these goals ensures a focused approach, helping individuals stay on track toward long-term financial stability.

Identifying financial goals marks the beginning of the journey toward financial literacy. It's important to distinguish between short-term and long-term objectives, as this differentiation helps clarify priorities and maintain focus. Short-term goals might include saving for a vacation or a gadget, while long-term aspirations could involve buying a house or planning for retirement. Each type of goal requires different strategies and timelines. For instance, when you're saving for a short-term goal, you may use a savings account for quick access and low risk. In contrast, long-term goals might involve investments like stocks or bonds, which typically offer higher returns over time but come with greater risk.

Setting goals also means they should be realistic. There's little sense in aiming to save an unrealistic amount if your current income does not support it. Instead, by understanding what is achievable, you maintain motivation and avoid frustration. Ensuring relevance keeps your goals aligned with your personal values and long-term vision, making decisions like prioritizing debt repayment over luxury purchases more straightforward. Lastly, setting time-bound goals establishes a sense of urgency, encouraging consistent effort and preventing procrastination. This structured timeframe also provides opportunities for regular reviews and adjustments, ensuring accountability for progress (*SMART Goals*, n.d.).

Once goals are identified and SMART criteria applied, developing an actionable plan becomes essential. This involves breaking down larger aspirations into smaller, manageable tasks. For example, if your goal is to travel abroad, an actionable plan would include steps such as setting monthly savings targets, researching costs, booking in advance, and adjusting spending habits. These tangible actions make daunting goals feel less overwhelming and more achievable.

An actionable financial plan also includes creating a budget to track income and expenses relative to each goal. Budgeting allows for intentional decision-making regarding spending, saving, and investing, ensuring that each financial choice contributes to achieving your set objectives. Consider using tools like spreadsheets or apps designed to help categorize expenses and visualize budget adherence. Consistent monitoring of your budget underscores accountability, which reinforces discipline and enhances the prospects of success.

Important to maintaining progress is regular monitoring, the final step in successfully achieving financial goals. Monitoring progress entails evaluating how well you're sticking to your plan and meeting your benchmarks. Regularly reviewing your progress allows you to identify areas that may require adjustment, whether it's refining your savings plan or reassessing your investment decisions. This ongoing attention helps maintain discipline, prevents stagnation, and ensures continued momentum toward achieving your financial goals.

Additionally, maintaining accountability is crucial for meeting financial goals. Sharing your goals with a trusted friend or financial advisor can provide added motivation and support. Having someone to report to regularly offers external encouragement to remain committed, and they can offer constructive feedback when needed.

Make sure you also take time to celebrate successes along this journey. Recognizing when you've achieved a milestone or reached a goal boosts morale and cultivates a positive mindset toward further achievements. Each celebration signifies progress and serves as a reminder of what disciplined financial management can accomplish. Whether it's a small congratulatory treat or a public acknowledgment of your success, celebrating victories keeps enthusiasm high.

Steering clear of common mistakes is just as important. Often, individuals set themselves up for disappointment by setting unrealistic goals without considering their current financial situation. To avoid this, it's essential to review your budget first and begin with goals that are achievable. Establishing smaller, initial milestones creates a strong base for progressively working toward more ambitious targets.

Having a clear plan is indispensable. Without an actionable trajectory, even the best-laid goals risk stagnation. Establish strategies and consider potential setbacks to ensure flexibility in adapting plans without deviating from the goal. Tracking progress consistently via varied methods—whether through apps or notebooks—ensures alignment with your aspirations and timely recognition of hurdles.

Numerous tools are available to assist in tracking and managing your financial goals. Apps and online platforms offer features like reminders, progress charts, and personalized insights, which simplify the process and enhance motivation. These resources provide a clear visual of your progress, helping you stay organized and make adjustments as needed. By offering real-time updates, they enable you to stay focused and adaptable, ensuring you're consistently working toward your financial objectives.

AVOIDING DEBT PITFALLS

Understanding debt is an essential aspect of financial literacy, as it enables you to make well-informed borrowing decisions that are important for maintaining financial independence. Debt can take various forms, each with its own set of characteristics and consequences. For example, student loans often come with lower interest rates and flexible repayment options, making them easier to manage compared to credit card debt, which typically carries high interest rates and severe penalties for missed payments. Mortgages, or home loans, are another form of debt, typically seen as more manageable due to their secured nature. However, they require a clear understanding of long-term commitments and the way interest accumulates over time. Recognizing the differences between these types of debt helps individuals approach borrowing with greater insight and planning.

High-interest debt, particularly from credit cards, can become a significant burden if not managed properly. Credit cards often entice users with the promise of buying now and paying later, but this convenience comes at a steep price if balances are not paid in full every month. Awareness of the impact of such debt is vital for making better financial decisions. For instance, understanding that minimum payments mostly cover interest rather than reducing principal debt is critical. This realization prompts individuals to explore alternative solutions, like consolidating debts or seeking lower-interest financing options. Consolidation loans, for instance, allow borrowers to combine multiple debts into a single payment plan, often at a lower interest rate, simplifying the repayment process.

Engaging in practical debt management strategies is key to prioritizing repayment and achieving financial stability. Creating a detailed repayment plan is an effective strategy. This involves listing all existing debts along with their interest rates and monthly obligations. Once this is outlined, focusing on high-interest debts first—often referred to as the "debt avalanche" method—can save money in the long run by reducing overall interest payments. Automating payments ensures consistency and prevents missed deadlines, which could otherwise lead to additional charges and negatively impact credit scores.

Another strategic approach is implementing the "debt snowball" method, where smaller debts are paid off first to build momentum. This psychological win boosts morale and motivation, encouraging continued adherence to the repayment plan. Setting aside extra funds or windfalls, such as tax refunds or bonuses, specifically for debt payments, accelerates the path to becoming debt-free. It's vital to keep an eye on spending habits closely, ensuring that unnecessary expenditures are curbed to align with financial goals.

Developing healthy credit habits is vital for lowering borrowing costs and unlocking future opportunities. A good credit score is vital to this process, as it is determined by factors such as your debt history, repayment behavior, and credit utilization ratios. Maintaining a strong credit score enables access to better interest rates and loan terms. Simple actions like maintaining low credit card balances, paying bills on time, and avoiding unnecessary credit lines can all boost your credit score. Even after clearing debts, regularly monitoring your credit report helps protect against identity theft and errors that could negatively affect your financial standing.

Introducing automation tools, budgeting apps, or online financial planners can help reinforce these concepts by keeping you organized and committed to your financial goals. These tools provide detailed insights into your spending and offer real-time alerts, which can help you track expenses and avoid overspending, a common cause of debt. Additionally, credit counseling services provide personalized guidance for those needing assistance in managing their finances more effectively.

Being proactive about managing debts and building robust credit habits paves the way for a secure financial future. Armed with knowledge and well-defined action strategies, individuals gain the ability to make informed decisions, reducing dependence on borrowed funds while enhancing opportunities for wealth building (*10 Strategies to Avoid Getting into Debt*, n.d.; Morgan, 2024).

IMPORTANCE OF FINANCIAL EDUCATION

The need for financial education has never been more important, especially for children as they learn to navigate complex financial systems. It is essential for educators and parents to instill financial literacy in children early, as it equips them with the knowledge and skills necessary to make informed choices in the future. With access to credit and investment opportunities on the rise, individuals are faced with numerous decisions that can affect their financial well-being. Financial education lays the groundwork for this understanding, empowering children to approach these decisions with confidence and ultimately promoting financial security and independence throughout their lives.

Financial education raises awareness about essential money management techniques. Grasping the fundamentals of budgeting, saving, investing, and debt management provides individuals with the essential tools to make informed financial decisions. For example, mastering the art of creating and sticking to a budget enables individuals to manage their income effectively, ensuring they can cover immediate needs while also saving for future goals. This foundational knowledge can prevent many common pitfalls associated with poor money management, such as accumulating unnecessary debt or failing to save for emergencies.

Financial education encourages responsible financial behavior and decision-making. Understanding financial principles such as interest rates, inflation, and risk management helps individuals assess the potential outcomes of their financial decisions. People who are financially literate are better equipped to weigh the pros and cons of taking on debt, investing in certain assets, or making large purchases. This discernment is essential for fostering positive financial habits that pave the way for a stable economic future.

One of the key benefits of increased financial knowledge is the boost in confidence it provides individuals when handling finances. Many people feel overwhelmed by the complexity of personal finance, which can lead to anxiety and stress. However, when individuals have a solid grasp of financial concepts, they feel more empowered to manage their money effectively and take control of their financial future. They are more likely to engage in proactive behaviors such as regularly reviewing their financial statements, comparing financial products before making a purchase, and seeking advice when necessary.

Ongoing education and the ability to adapt to financial shifts are vital for improving financial literacy. The financial landscape is constantly shifting due to technological advancements, regulatory changes, and global economic fluctuations. As such, staying updated on these changes is important in maintaining financial stability. For example, the rise of digital banking and cryptocurrencies has introduced new opportunities and risks that require careful consideration. Committing to continuous learning in finance allows individuals to better anticipate and adapt to changes, thereby maintaining their financial resilience.

Financial education also extends its benefits beyond individual gains, contributing to broader societal well-being. A financially literate population is more likely to engage in behaviors that promote economic growth and stability. For example, financially educated individuals are more likely to save for retirement, reducing the strain on public pension systems. They are also more inclined to invest in businesses and innovations, driving economic development and job creation. A society that values financial literacy fosters an environment where individuals feel supported in their financial endeavors, leading to decreased inequality and increased social mobility.

The positive impact of financial education is well-documented. Studies have shown that participation in financial literacy programs leads to improved financial outcomes, such as higher savings rates, reduced debt levels, and increased participation in retirement plans (*Benefits of Financial Education,* n.d.). These benefits highlight the importance of integrating financial education into various aspects of life, including schools, workplaces, and community programs. Ensuring that financial education is accessible and inclusive enables individuals from diverse backgrounds to gain the skills necessary for achieving financial independence.

Implementing financial education initiatives should be a priority for governments, educational institutions, and organizations. Parents and educators can significantly contribute to the development and support of these programs through their active involvement. Programs tailored to specific demographics, such as teens and young adults, can address the unique challenges and opportunities faced by different groups. For example, educational programs targeted at young adults could cover topics like managing student loans, understanding credit scores, and planning for long-term financial goals. Involving parents in discussions about financial literacy and encouraging educators to incorporate financial topics into the curriculum can create a supportive environment. These targeted strategies help ensure that financial education is both relevant and effective.

Additionally, leveraging technology can enhance the reach and effectiveness of financial education. Online platforms, apps, and interactive tools provide engaging and convenient ways for individuals to learn about personal finance. These resources can offer personalized feedback and simulate real-life financial scenarios, allowing users to practice decision-making in a low-risk environment. Leveraging technology makes financial education more dynamic and better suited to the needs of learners.

HOW TECHNOLOGY HELPS TEENAGERS LEARN ABOUT MONEY

Financial literacy is one of the most important life skills a teenager can develop, yet it's rarely emphasized in traditional education. As teens start earning money from part-time jobs or receiving allowances, they often face real-world financial decisions without the knowledge to navigate them. Fortunately, technology is stepping in to fill the gap. Today's teens have access to a wide variety of tools—like mobile apps and interactive calculators—that make learning about money not only easier but also engaging, personalized, and fun. These tools provide teens with the opportunity to develop strong money habits early, setting the stage for confident, informed financial decision-making in adulthood.

EveryDollar

EveryDollar is a budgeting app based on zero-based budgeting, a method where users assign every dollar of their income to a specific purpose. Designed to encourage proactive financial planning, the app is straightforward: Teens input how much money they have—whether from a job, allowance, or gifts—and then allocate it to categories like saving, spending, and giving. The app helps users see how much they've planned versus how much they've actually spent, encouraging adjustments when needed. Manual entry is free, while the premium version connects to bank accounts and tracks transactions automatically.

BENEFITS

- teaches the concept of zero-based budgeting and intentional money use
- builds awareness of where money is going and how to plan for expenses
- encourages decision-making by helping teens prioritize spending
- reinforces financial responsibility and discipline over time
- offers real-world practice in managing and adjusting a monthly budget

Zogo

Zogo is a financial education app designed specifically for teens and young adults. It breaks down complex financial topics, such as budgeting, credit, investing, and taxes, into short, gamified lessons. Each topic is taught through modules followed by quizzes. Completing modules earns users "pineapples," which can be redeemed for gift cards. With its interactive, reward-based system, Zogo keeps users motivated while they learn.

BENEFITS

- covers a broad range of financial topics in an engaging format
- encourages retention with short quizzes and instant feedback
- makes financial literacy fun and accessible for all skill levels
- reinforces key concepts through repetition and gamified incentives
- builds real-world understanding of critical money topics teens will face

YNAB (You Need A Budget)

YNAB is a budgeting app that focuses on forward-thinking financial planning. Instead of budgeting monthly, YNAB teaches users to budget only the money they currently have, encouraging them to allocate funds with intention. The app provides educational videos, workshops, and resources to help teens build smart habits. YNAB emphasizes flexibility and control—if users overspend in one category, they learn to adjust by pulling from another.

BENEFITS

- promotes adaptive, real-time budgeting and planning
- reinforces prioritization and adjusting to changing needs
- builds financial awareness through hands-on decision-making
- includes built-in learning resources for a deeper understanding
- develops proactive money habits and long-term thinking

GoHenry

GoHenry combines a prepaid debit card for teens with a financial education app. Parents can load money onto the card and assign it to different purposes, such as spending, saving, or giving. Teens use the app to manage their money and complete educational "money missions" on budgeting, saving, and financial responsibility. Parents receive real-time updates and can set spending limits, allowing for guided independence.

BENEFITS

- combines real-life practice with built-in learning modules
- teaches the basics of earning, saving, and budgeting through experience
- provides a safe environment to learn from financial choices
- encourages responsibility and financial independence
- opens up structured family conversations about money

Bankaroo

Bankaroo is a virtual banking app that allows kids and teens to simulate managing money. It enables users to track virtual income, set budgets, and allocate money toward different savings goals. Since no real money is involved, it's a low-pressure environment to build core financial skills. Parents or teachers can add virtual deposits, and teens manually log "purchases" to reflect spending.

BENEFITS

- teaches basic financial literacy in a safe, controlled space
- encourages saving, planning, and budgeting without real-world risk
- builds early confidence with money management concepts
- ideal for preteens just beginning to understand finances
- promotes independence and goal-oriented thinking

HowTheMarketWorks

HowTheMarketWorks is a stock market simulation platform that lets teens invest virtual money in real-time markets. Users get a fake portfolio—usually $100,000—to buy and sell stocks, build strategies, and track performance. The platform includes lessons on investing, risk management, diversification, and economic indicators. It's widely used in schools and investment clubs to teach the fundamentals of trading and long-term growth.

BENEFITS

- demonstrates how investing works through simulation
- teaches risk-taking, strategy, and market analysis without financial loss
- encourages critical thinking and economic awareness
- supports learning through experimentation and reflection
- helps teens explore investing before using real money

NerdWallet's Credit Score Simulator

NerdWallet's Credit Score Simulator lets users see how different actions— like paying off debt, missing a payment, or opening a credit card—would impact a credit score. Although teens may not yet have a credit score, this tool helps them understand how financial behavior affects future borrowing power. It's interactive and visual, showing estimated score changes based on simulated decisions.

BENEFITS

- explains how credit scores are calculated and influenced
- helps teens understand the consequences of borrowing behaviors
- builds knowledge before they enter the credit system

- encourages good habits like on-time payments and avoiding unnecessary debt
- provides a risk-free way to explore how credit works

Goodbudget

Goodbudget is a digital envelope budgeting app that helps users plan and track their spending. Instead of linking directly to bank accounts, users manually allocate funds into virtual "envelopes" for categories like groceries, rent, or entertainment. This method encourages intentional spending and proactive financial planning.

BENEFITS

- teaches disciplined, category-based budgeting using the envelope method
- encourages mindful spending by requiring manual transaction entries
- facilitates shared budgeting among family members or partners
- provides a clear, straightforward interface without unnecessary distractions
- helps users prioritize expenses based on personal values and goals

PocketGuard

PocketGuard is a budgeting app designed to simplify money management by showing users how much disposable income they have after accounting for bills, goals, and necessities. By linking to financial accounts, it automatically categorizes expenses and tracks spending in real time. The app also offers features like subscription tracking and a debt payoff plan.

BENEFITS

- provides a clear overview of available funds to prevent overspending
- automates expense categorization and tracks spending habits
- identifies recurring subscriptions and helps manage or cancel them
- offers tools to create and follow a personalized debt repayment plan
- supports goal setting and monitors progress toward financial objectives

Honeydue

Honeydue is a financial app designed for couples to manage their money together. It allows partners to link accounts, set budgets, track expenses, and communicate about finances within the app. Users can choose what information to share, promoting transparency and collaboration without compromising privacy.

BENEFITS

- facilitates open financial communication between partners
- allows customizable sharing settings for individual and joint accounts
- provides bill reminders to avoid missed payments
- enables in-app messaging to discuss transactions and budgets
- helps couples align their financial goals and spending habits

Empower

Empower is a comprehensive financial app that combines budgeting tools with features like automated savings, investment tracking, and financial goal setting. It offers a holistic view of users' financial health by aggregating various accounts and providing insights into spending patterns. Additionally, Empower provides cash advances to help cover unexpected expenses.

BENEFITS

- aggregates multiple financial accounts for a unified overview
- assists in setting and tracking personalized financial goals
- offers automated savings features to encourage consistent saving habits
- provides investment tracking to monitor portfolio performance
- delivers cash advances up to $300 without credit checks or interest

Credit Karma

Credit Karma is a free financial app that offers users access to their credit scores, credit reports, and personalized recommendations for financial products. It also provides tools like a credit score simulator, identity monitoring, and financial calculators to help users understand and improve their financial standing.

BENEFITS

- provides free access to credit scores and reports from major bureaus
- offers personalized insights and recommendations to improve credit health
- includes a credit score simulator to predict the impact of financial decisions

- monitors for identity theft and alerts users to potential breaches
- helps users find and compare financial products tailored to their profiles

Emma

Emma is a money management app that connects to users' bank accounts to provide real-time insights into spending, budgeting, and saving. It identifies subscriptions, tracks expenses, and offers tools to set budgets and financial goals. Emma also includes features like cashback offers and rent reporting to credit bureaus.

BENEFITS

- aggregates multiple accounts for a comprehensive financial overview
- automatically detects and tracks recurring subscriptions
- provides budgeting tools and spending analysis to promote financial awareness
- offers cashback deals to help users save on purchases
- reports rent payments to credit bureaus to assist in building credit history

An Example of the Importance of Financial Education

When Alex was growing up, her parents didn't teach her much about money. She knew how to spend it, but didn't understand how to manage it. As a teenager, Alex got her first part-time job and was excited to earn her own income. However, when she went to spend it, she quickly realized that she didn't have a plan for it. She would buy clothes, hang out with friends, and not think much about the future. Eventually, she found herself with little to no savings, and her checking account balance was lower than expected. She didn't know how to budget, save, or manage her money in a way that would set her up for success.

It wasn't until Alex began college that she learned the importance of financial education. Her school offered workshops on budgeting, saving, and managing expenses, and she decided to attend one. That workshop completely changed her perspective on money. She learned how to track her spending, start saving—even if it was just a small amount—and avoid unnecessary spending. Alex began applying these lessons in her everyday life, and over time, she developed financial habits that helped her make smarter decisions. She realized that financial education isn't just about knowing how to spend; it's about making informed choices that ensure long-term financial success.

This knowledge helped Alex to take control of her finances and gave her confidence in her ability to make smart financial decisions. Looking back, she recognizes the importance of teaching these skills to young people early on. Had she understood these concepts as a child or teen, she would have been better prepared to handle her money and make informed choices much sooner.

Financial education is something that everyone should have access to—whether through parents, educators, or community programs—so that future generations can avoid the stress and uncertainty that come with poor financial management.

KEY TAKEAWAYS

- Understanding financial concepts is essential for achieving peace of mind, as it enables individuals to make informed choices about managing their money.

- Being familiar with basic financial terms like income, expenses, assets, and liabilities is key to managing money effectively and making sound financial decisions.

- Effective budgeting helps allocate money toward key areas such as housing (25%–35%), insurance (10%–20%), food (10%–15%), and savings (10%–15%).

- Budgeting for giving back (10%–15%) and personal expenses (5%–10%) fosters financial responsibility and self-care.

- Developing a savings habit, setting achievable financial goals, and using automated savings systems can provide financial security and prepare individuals for unexpected costs.

- Recognizing different types of debt and adopting strategies such as the debt avalanche or snowball methods can reduce financial strain and support long-term stability.

- Early and ongoing financial education provides individuals with the knowledge needed to make informed choices, fostering responsible financial behavior and improving overall financial health.

- Staying informed about changes in the financial landscape through ongoing learning helps individuals stay resilient and adapt to new challenges.

- Building a supportive network and utilizing tools like budgeting apps and financial literacy programs can enhance financial education and promote better money management.

- By improving financial literacy and applying effective budgeting and saving techniques, individuals can move toward financial independence, reducing stress and creating opportunities for a more fulfilling future.

CONTINUE YOUR JOURNEY OF LETTING GO

You don't have to walk this path alone.

To help you begin with gentleness and courage, I've created something special to walk beside you: a companion to guide you through this journey of healing and release.

To support you along the way, you'll receive access to the **Free Companion Course**: *Breathe, Release, Restore: 7 Days to Emotional Healing and Inner Peace.*

Scan the QR code to unlock your free course.

This guided 7-day experience brings the lessons from this book to life through:

- **Mindful breathing practices** to calm your body and mind.
- **Gentle yoga and reflection** to release stored emotions.
- **Movement-based mindfulness** to embody what you learn and restore balance.

Each day helps you embody what you've read—**turning awareness into action** and **action into transformation**.

Breathe in peace.
Release what no longer serves you.
Restore your strength.

Acknowledgments

This book is the culmination of personal and professional experiences that have shaped my journey of learning to release past pain and trauma, and embracing the freedom of new beginnings. Writing these pages has been both a healing process and a privilege, and I feel deeply honored to be able to reach out to teens, parents, educators, and healers who may find strength and encouragement within these words.

I owe my deepest gratitude to my parents, whose love and values laid the foundation for my resilience, and to my sisters, whose presence has been a constant source of comfort and inspiration. To my children, who continue to remind me of the beauty of growth, change, and unconditional love—you are my greatest teachers. I am equally grateful to my close friends and to the many special people who have crossed my path, each leaving behind valuable lessons and encouragement that have helped me grow.

This book would not have been possible without the wisdom, support, and kindness of all those who believed in me and inspired me to persevere. Your faith has fueled my passion to share this message of healing and hope with others.

From the depths of my heart, I am genuinely and forever grateful.

References

Ackerman, C. (2017, March 20). *25 CBT techniques and worksheets for cognitive behavioral therapy*. Positive Psychology. https://positivepsychology.com/cbt-cognitive-behavioral-therapy-techniques-worksheets/

All you need to know about healthy relationships. (n.d.). *Mind and Body Counseling Services.* https://mindbodycounselingreno.com/blog/relationships/all-you-need-to-know-about-healthy-relationships/

Andrews, A. J. (2024, September 17). *How to embrace mindfulness: A guide to living in the moment.* Medium. https://medium.com/zone-of-freedom/how-to-embrace-mindfulness-a-guide-to-living-in-the-moment-95e0362ca7e2

Aquin, J. P., El-Gabalawy, R., Sala, T., & Sareen, J. (2017). Anxiety disorders and general medical conditions: Current research and future directions. *American Psychiatric Publishing, 15*(2), 173–181. https://doi.org/10.1176/appi.focus.20160044

Arnsten, A., Mazure, C. M., & Sinha, R. (2012). This is your brain in meltdown. *Scientific American, 306*(4), 48–53. https://doi.org/10.1038/scientificamerican0412-48

Benefits of financial education: Financial literacy benefits. (n.d.). NFEC. https://www.financialeducatorscouncil.org/benefits-of-financial-education/

BetterHelp Editorial Team. (2025, February 28). *Impacts of social pressure.* BetterHelp. https://www.betterhelp.com/advice/general/how-does-social-pressure-impact-our-choices/

Budgeting basics: The 50-30-20 rule. (n.d.). United Nations Federal Credit Union. https://www.unfcu.org/financial-wellness/50-30-20-rule/

Carter, S. (2024, July 10). *25 grounding techniques to support mental wellness*. All Points North. https://apn.com/resources/25-grounding-techniques-to-support-mental-wellness/

CFI Team. (n.d.). *Financial literacy*. Corporate Finance Institute. https://corporatefinanceinstitute.com/resources/wealth-management/financial-literacy/

Chae, C. (2024, June 13). Building healthy friendships. *Abundance Therapy Center*. https://www.abundancetherapycenter.com/blog/building-healthy-friendships

CounselorAid. (2024, November 8). DBT emotion regulation skills for managing workplace stress. https://counseloraid.com/dbt-emotion-regulation-skills-for-managing-workplace-stress/

Craft, L. L., & Perna, F. M. (2004, June 1). The benefits of exercise for the clinically depressed. *The Primary Care Companion to the Journal of Clinical Psychiatry*, *06*(03), 104–111. https://doi.org/10.4088/pcc.v06n0301

Cuncic, A. (2024, February 12). *Seven active listening techniques for better communication*. Verywell Mind. http://www.verywellmind.com/what-is-active-listening-3024343

Elise, C. (2019, November 10). *Rituals for letting go*. Medium. https://medium.com/@septemberstar/rituals-for-letting-go-910b6a933689

Empowering students with assertiveness skills. (n.d.). Care Clinics. https://care-clinics.com/empowering-students-with-assertiveness-skills/

Fernando, J. (2024, June 7). *Financial literacy: What it is, and why it is so important*. Investopedia. https://www.investopedia.com/terms/f/financial-literacy.asp

5 conflict resolution strategies for the workplace. (2024, December 17). *Champlain College Online*. https://online.champlain.edu/blog/top-conflict-resolution-strategies

5 ways stress can impact your memory (and what to do about it). (n.d.). *Calm Blog*. https://www.calm.com/blog/stress-and-memory

Godwin, J. (2023, March 12). *Let's talk about... individuality.* Let's Talk about Mental Health. https://letstalkaboutmentalhealth.com.au/2023/03/12/individuality/

Guide to developing a growth mindset. (2024, December 16). Tavahealth. https://www.tavahealth.com/resources/guide-growth-mindset

Hancock, J. (n.d.). *What are your values?.* Mind Tools. https://www.mindtools.com/a5eygum/what-are-your-values

Holland, K. (2025, April 18). *Amygdala hijack: When emotion takes over.* Healthline. https://www.healthline.com/health/stress/amygdala-hijack

How can we protect, promote, and maintain body image? Mental Health Foundation. https://www.mentalhealth.org.uk/our-work/research/body-image-how-we-think-and-feel-about-our-bodies/how-can-we-protect-promote-and-maintain-body-image

How the outdoors can improve your mood. (2024, April 9). Cleveland Clinic. https://newsroom.clevelandclinic.org/2024/04/09/how-the-outdoors-can-improve-your-mood

How to embrace self-acceptance and cultivate self-compassion. (n.d.). Changes Big and Small. https://changesbigandsmall.com/how-to-embrace-self-acceptance-and-cultivate-self-compassion/

How to foster a growth mindset in the classroom. (2020, December 10). School of Education. *American University.* https://soeonline.american.edu/blog/growth-mindset-in-the-classroom/

How to handle peer pressure. (n.d.). Fairfax County Public Schools. https://www.fcps.edu/student-wellness-tips/peer-pressure

Howards, Y. (2024, August 19). The power of forgiveness in emotional healing. *Brighter Tomorrow Counseling Services.* https://brightertomorrowtherapy.com/power-of-forgiveness/.

Hurley, K. (2024, July 29). *Resilience: A guide to facing life's challenges, adversities, and crises.* Everyday Health. https://www.everydayhealth.com/wellness/resilience/

Hypothalamic-pituitary-adrenal (HPA) axis. (2024, April 12). Cleveland Clinic. https://my.clevelandclinic.org/health/body/hypothalamic-pituitary-adrenal-hpa-axis

The importance of boundaries for your mental well-being: From a Birmingham therapist. (n.d.). Empower Counseling & Coaching. https://empowercounselingllc.com/the-importance-of-boundaries-for-your-mental-wellbeing/

Insight Timer Editorial Team. (n.d.). Top 10 mindfulness grounding techniques for stress-resilient professionals. *Insight Timer Blog.* https://insighttimer.com/blog/mindfulness-grounding-techniques-for-professionals/

Kohrt, B. A., Ottman, K., Panter-Brick, C., Konner, M., & Patel, V. (2020). Why we heal: The evolution of psychological healing and implications for global mental health. *Clinical Psychology Review, 82*(82). https://doi.org/10.1016/j.cpr.2020.101920

Lee, R. (n.d.). *The power of forgiveness in emotional healing.* Families. https://vocal.media/families/the-power-of-forgiveness-in-emotional-healing

Lumley, M. A., Cohen, J. L., Borszcz, G. S., Cano, A., Radcliffe, A. M., Porter, L. S., Schubiner, H., & Keefe, F. J. (2011). Pain and emotion: A biopsychosocial review of recent research. *Journal of Clinical Psychology, 67*(9), 942–968. https://doi.org/10.1002/jclp.20816

Mayer, H. (2023, July 3). *The art of self-compassion: A journey to mental well-being and self-improvement.* Inner Space Counselling. https://innerspacecounselling.com.au/the-art-of-self-compassion-a-journey-to-mental-well-being-and-self-improvement/

Mayo Clinic Staff. (2022, October 11). *Mindfulness exercises.* Mayo Clinic. https://www.mayoclinic.org/healthy-lifestyle/consumer-health/in-depth/mindfulness-exercises/art-20046356

Mayo Clinic Staff. (2025, March 27). *Support groups: Make connections, get help.* Mayo Clinic. https://www.mayoclinic.org/healthy-lifestyle/stress-management/in-depth/support-groups/art-20044655

McEwen, B. S. (2017). Neurobiological and systemic effects of chronic stress. *Chronic Stress, 1*(1). https://doi.org/10.1177/2470547017692328

Michot, E. (2023). *The role of societal expectations in the development of self-critical tendencies*. Academia. https://www.academia.edu/104726604/The_Role_Of_Societal_Expectations_In_The_Development_Of_Self_Critical_Tendencies

Mindfulness meditation: Types, strategies & benefits. (2024, June 10). *Bloomington Meadows Hospital.* https://bloomingtonmeadows.com/blog/mindfulness-meditation-types-strategies-benefits/

Mindfulness techniques for better mental health. (n.d.) *Hope Mountain Behavioral Health.* https://www.myhopemountain.org/blog/mindfulness-techniques-for-better-mental-health

Modern Recovery Editorial Team. (2023, July 6). *Emotional expression: Definition, benefits & techniques.* https://modernrecoveryservices.com/wellness/coping/skills/emotional/emotional-expression/

Morgan. L. (2024, December 4). 5 ways to avoid common debt pitfalls with smart financial tools. *Morgan & Morgan.* https://morganlawyers.com/5-ways-to-avoid-common-debt-pitfalls-with-smart-financial-tools/

National Institutes of Health. (n.d.). *Emotional wellness toolkit.* https://www.nih.gov/health-information/emotional-wellness-toolkit

Norelli, S. K., Long, A., & Krepps, J. M. (2023, August 28). *Relaxation Techniques*. StatPearls Publishing. https://www.ncbi.nlm.nih.gov/books/NBK513238/

Overcoming obstacles: Strategies for resilience and adaptability. (n.d.). Think Coaching Academy. https://www.thinkcoachingacademy.co.za/overcoming-obstacles-strategies-for-resilience-and-adaptability/

Pederson, L. (2019, October 17). Mindfulness exercises: 73 ways to practice the. technique. *The MHS Journals.* https://www.mhs-dbt.com/blog/mindfulness-exercises/

Peer pressure or influence: Pre-teens and teenagers. (2024, May 8). Raising Children Network. https://raisingchildren.net.au/teens/behaviour/peers-friends-trends/peer-influence

Pennock, S. F. (2024, October 31). Understanding the importance of embracing your true self in authenticity coaching. *Quenza.* https://quenza.com/blog/embracing-your-true-self/

Perry, E. (2023, August 8). The meaning of personal values: How they shape your life. *Betterup.* https://www.betterup.com/blog/meaning-of-personal-values

Perry, E. (2024, March 26). 33 self-esteem journal prompts for confidence & self-compassion. *Betterup.* https://www.betterup.com/blog/self-esteem-journal-prompts

Peterson, M. (2023, May 25). The lingering burden: Exploring the long-term effects of stress on mental wellness and its impact on a person's life. *Balanced Spine Center.* https://balancedspinecenter.com/blog/the-lingering-burden-exploring-the-long-term-effects-of-stress-on-mental-wellness-and-its-impact-on-a-person-s-life

Purdue Global. (2024, January 10). How to set professional goals for yourself. *Purdue Global.* https://www.purdueglobal.edu/blog/careers/setting-professional-goals-with-examples/

Raising empathetic children: Building a more inclusive society. London Governess. https://londongoverness.com/raising-empathetic-children-building-a-more-inclusive-society/

Raypole, C. (2025, May 28). *How to hack your hormones for a better mood.* Healthline. https://www.healthline.com/health/happy-hormone

Riess, H. (2017). The science of empathy. *Journal of Patient Experience, 4*(2), 74–77. https://doi.org/10.1177/2374373517699267

Robinson, L., Segal, J., & Smith, M. (2025, March 13). *Effective communication: Improving your interpersonal skills.* Help Guide. https://www.helpguide.org/relationships/communication/effective-communication

Schmitz, T. (2016, June 3). *The importance of emotional awareness in communication*. The Conover Company. https://www.conovercompany.com/the-importance-of-emotional-awareness-in-communication/

Setting SMART financial goals. (2024, July 31). *Desert Financial*. https://www.desertfinancial.com/en/learn/blog/financial-education/smart-goals

7 calming yoga poses for stress relief. (2024, June 11). *Palladium Private*. https://www.palladiumprivate.com/blog/7-yoga-poses-for-stress-relief/

Shonk, K. (2025, May 25). *3 negotiation strategies for conflict resolution*. Harvard Law School. https://www.pon.harvard.edu/daily/dispute-resolution/3-negotiation-strategies-for-conflict-resolution/

SMART goals. (n.d.). Khan Academy. https://www.khanacademy.org/college-careers-more/financial-literacy/xa6995ea67a8e9fdd:financial-goals/xa6995ea67a8e9fdd:smart-goals/a/smart-goals

Stef, S. (2023, November 26). *Effective communication skills: Tips for active listening, assertiveness, conflict resolution, and conflict resolution, and fostering healthy relationships*. Medium. https://medium.com/@stellafong/effective-communication-skills-tips-for-active-listening-assertiveness-conflict-resolution-and-2dcdf6430ace

Sutton, J. (2018, May 14). *5 benefits of journaling for mental health*. Positive Psychology. https://positivepsychology.com/benefits-of-journaling/

Taylor, D. (2023, July 28). Active listening and empathy for better working relationships. *Forbes*. https://www.forbes.com/councils/forbesbusinesscouncil/2023/07/28/active-listening-and-empathy-for-better-working-relationships/

10 effective strategies to manage overwhelming emotions. (n.d.). DBT of South Jersey. https://dbtofsouthjersey.com/how-to-manage-overwhelming-emotions/

10 strategies to avoid getting into debt. (n.d.). Central Bank. https://www.centralbank.net/learning-center/strategies-to-avoid-debt/

Tickner, A. (2024, November 4). Goal setting basics: Long-term and short-term goals for success. *Speexx*. https://www.speexx.com/speexx-blog/goal-setting-basics-long-term-and-short-term-goals-for-success/

United Way NCA. (2023, June 6). Youth financial literacy: Why is it important? *United Way of the National Capital Area*. https://unitedwaynca.org/blog/financial-literacy-for-youth/

wadmin. (2024a, February 16). *Emotional triggers: Why they matter & how to manage them effectively*. Mindful Health Solutions. https://mindfulhealthsolutions.com/emotional-triggers-why-they-matter-how-to-manage-them-effectively/

wadmin. (2024b, July 19). *Find your personal triggers in 7 simple steps and strengthen your mental health*. Mindful Health Solutions. https://mindfulhealthsolutions.com/find-your-personal-triggers-in-7-simple-steps/

wadmin. (2024c, August 9). *24 ways to transform negative thoughts with cognitive behavioral techniques*. Mindful Health Solutions. https://mindfulhealthsolutions.com/24-ways-to-transform-negative-thoughts-with-cognitive-behavioral-techniques/

Walsh, J. (2015, July 12). *The importance of creating our own rituals*. Jessica A. Walsh. https://www.jessicaannwalsh.com/2015/07/creating-rituals.html/

Whiteside, E. (2024, August 22). *The 50/30/20 Budget rule explained with examples*. Investopedia. https://www.investopedia.com/ask/answers/022916/what-502030-budget-rule.asp

Why body positivity is important. (2024, October 15). Blue Ridge Treatment. https://www.blueridgetreatment.com/post/why-body-positivity-is-important

Wondermed. (2023, October 17). 10 ways to incorporate mindfulness into your life. https://blog.wondermed.com/10-ways-to-incorporate-mindfulness/

Wright, K. W. (2023, June 2). Self-Reflection: 300+ powerful questions for turning inward. *Day One*. https://dayoneapp.com/blog/self-reflection/

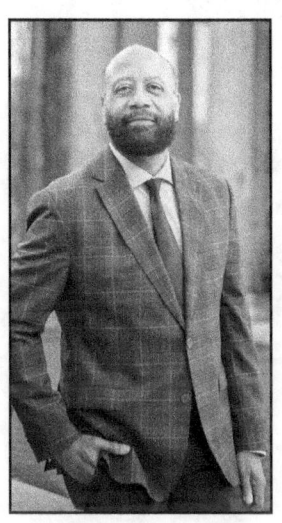

Dr. Jerome Puryear, MD, MBA, Dipl ABOM, is a physician, entrepreneur, and wellness advocate with over 25 years of experience helping people break free from stress, anxiety, and self-doubt. Drawing on his unique blend of medical expertise, business insight, and certification as a Duke-trained Health & Well-Being Coach, he empowers teens and young adults to release emotional burdens and live with greater clarity, resilience, and purpose. *Mastering the Art of Letting Go of Emotional Pain & Toxic Relationships* is his guide to building a healthier, more authentic life—starting from the inside out.

THANK YOU FOR READING

Your journey means so much.

If this book gave you hope, helped you let go,
or reminded you of your own strength,
I'd love to hear from you.

Please take a moment to leave a review on Amazon—
your words help this message reach others who need it too.

Scan the QR code below
to share your thoughts.

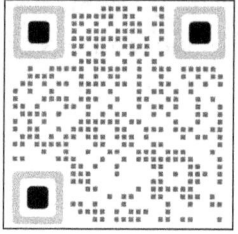

Your reflection might be exactly
what someone else needs
to start their healing journey.

www.ingramcontent.com/pod-product-compliance
Lightning Source LLC
Chambersburg PA
CBHW060416130626
46555CB00005B/2093

9798985996142